The British Veterinary
Profession, 1791 – 1948

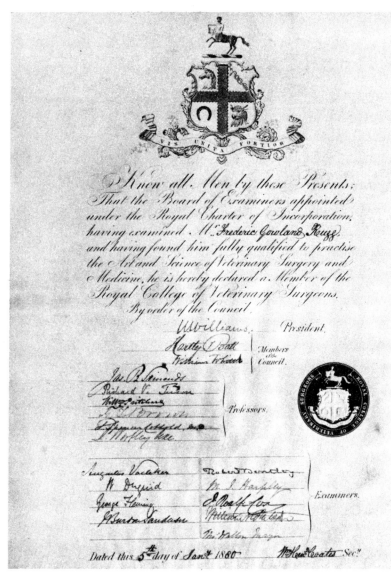

Certificate of Membership of
The Royal College of Veterinary Surgeons

PRESIDENT W. Williams. MEMBERS OF THE COUNCIL Hartley T. Batt, William Whittle. PROFESSORS Jas. B. Simonds, Richard V. Tuson, William Pritchard, G. T. Brown, T. Spencer Cobbold, M.D., J. Wortley Axe. EXAMINERS Augustus Voelcker, W. Duguid, George Fleming, J. Burdon Sanderson, Robert Bentley, M. J. Harpley, J. Roalfe Cox, William Robertson, Thos. Walton Mayer. Dated this 5th day of Jany. 1880 Wm. Henry Coates, SECRETARY.

IAIN PATTISON

The British Veterinary Profession
1791–1948

J.A.ALLEN

London

British Library Cataloguing in Publication Data

Pattison, Iain

The British veterinary profession 1791–1948
1. Veterinarians—Great Britain—History
I. Title
636.089′069   SF779.5

ISBN 0-85131-379-5

Published in 1984 in Great Britain by
J. A. Allen & Company Limited,
1, Lower Grosvenor Place,
Buckingham Palace Road,
London, SW1W 0EL.

© Iain Pattison 1984

Printed by Butler & Tanner Limited, Frome, Somerset.
Bound by WBC Bookbinders Limited, Maesteg, South Wales.

To

J.A.A.

whose interest in veterinary history

and personal generosity

made publication possible

Acknowledgements

The guidance of professional librarians was crucial in writing this book. Miss B. Horder and her staff at the Royal College of Veterinary Surgeons gave unstinted help, as did Mr R. Catton at The Royal Veterinary College. Miss Horder advised on preparation of the bibliography, and checked the references. The staff of the library of the Wellcome Institute for the History of Medicine assisted on many occasions.

The President and Council of The Royal College of Veterinary Surgeons, and Dr A.O. Betts, Principal of the Royal Veterinary College, kindly allowed unrestricted access to archives,

Mr M. Young and Mr P.G. Hignett, past Presidents of The Royal College of Veterinary Surgeons, and Mr C. Mitchell, lately editor of *The Veterinary Record*, gave valued advice on presentation of the manuscript.

The Wellcome Trust made a most generous contribution towards publication.

It is a pleasure to acknowledge so much help, from so many, so willingly given.

Contents

Illustrations

Author's Note

The similarity in titles of The Royal Veterinary College (the teaching school in London), and The Royal College of Veterinary Surgeons (the corporate and administrative body of the British veterinary profession) made it essential to modify one designation, so that each could easily be identified. The Royal Veterinary College has been called 'the London school,' therefore, and all other teaching colleges are referred to as schools. The Royal College of Veterinary Surgeons has been abbreviated to RCVS.

The National Veterinary Medical Association has been abbreviated to NVMA.

When this history was planned, it was decided to finish at a date approximately one generation earlier than the time of writing, for the reason that recent events cannot be assessed as objectively as those long past. The Veterinary Surgeons Act of 1948 separated two veterinary worlds, and that revolutionary legislation was a logical point at which to end the story.

CHAPTER 1

The beginning — A veterinary school for London in 1791

Veterinary surgeons were so named in 1796 by the British Army's Board of General Officers, to distinguish them from human surgeons. Previously they had been farriers. Before that, in the days of chivalry, they were marshals, and in Roman times they practised *medicina veterinaria* in a *veterinarium*.

The adjective 'veterinary' was popularised by Frenchman Charles Benôit Vial de St Bel (commonly called St Bel or Sainbel), whose Plan for "An Institution to Cultivate and Teach Veterinary Medicine" developed into Britain's first veterinary school, in London.

Animal-doctoring was 'farriery' before St Bel, but by the time the first diploma was granted from the London school in 1794, it described the holder as "qualified to practise the Veterinary Art."

What was this Art at the end of the eighteenth century?

Folk-lore and empiricism, especially in rural areas, with a whiff of rational husbandry. Great houses employed shoeing smiths and men with experience of livestock, especially of horses, and individual noblemen had veterinary advisers. Occasional writers of the period have left evidence of practical knowledge — James Clark, for example, Farrier to His Majesty for Scotland, whose "Treatise on the Prevention of Diseases Incidental to Horses" of 1788 has much sound sense.

But all too often treatment of animal ailments was born of ignorance so absolute that not only the disease but also the structure and working of the animal body were quite unknown. There was an ox, "labouring under hopeless constipation," to which was summoned "the old farrier or leech of the district. A cure was . . . confidently promised. A lively trout . . . was taken from the adjoining stream, and committed to the gullet of the patient, under the assurance that it would soon work its way through all impediments, and speedy relief be afforded." That neither ox nor trout survived was irrelevant. All had been done that could be done. Indeed, the most fortunate sick animals in the 18th century were those left untreated. Their companions, bled, purged, blistered, and fired, suffered and died.

There was great need for improvement in this Veterinary Art.

The world's first veterinary school was founded by Claude Bourgelat at Lyons in France in 1762. Other schools soon followed. In Britain, Edward Snape, Farrier to George III, established in 1778, in London, a "Hippiatric Infirmary for the instruction of pupils in the Profession," but the venture failed.

All credit for bringing to Britain the French idea of veterinary education, belongs to the Agricultural Society of Odiham in Hampshire. At a meeting of the Society in August 1785 it was agreed: "That Farriery is a most useful science and intimately connected with the Interests of Agriculture; that it is in a very imperfect neglected state and highly deserving the attention of all friends of Agricultural economy." Some three years later, having in the meantime collected the necessary funds, the Society arranged to send two or more boys to study at the veterinary school at Alfort near Paris. However, in 1789, before arrangements had been made to dispatch the young men to France, a member of the Odiham Society, Granville Penn, happened to meet M. St Bel, a French veterinarian and graduate of the Lyons school, who was visiting England. St Bel discussed with Penn a Plan for a veterinary school that he had canvassed unsuccessfully in France, and more recently in England. Penn was impressed. He helped St Bel to modify the Plan to suit conditions in England, and the result was a remarkable document that envisaged the organisation and administration of an institution that became the prototype for future British veterinary schools. It even suggested that the school should eventually be incorporated by Charter as "The Royal Veterinary College."

Backed by the Odiham Society, Penn set about obtaining financial support for a veterinary school in London. A London Committee of the Society was formed, meeting for the first time in November 1790 at the Prince of Wales Coffee House. The interest of wealthy and influential patrons made it possible for the London Committee at a meeting on 11th February 1791 to reaffirm its faith in: "The Benefits which must result from an Institution to cultivate and teach Veterinary Medicine," and on 18th February 1791 it adopted the name: "The Veterinary College, London." The Odiham Society withdrew from the scene, without rancour, so that matters in London could proceed independently.

St Bel was appointed Professor of the College. The choice was not surprising. Not only had the original Plan been his, but his veterinary experience was far wider than that of anyone in Britain.

The envisaged high status of the proposed veterinary school in London may be gauged from the fact that in March 1791 Sir George Baker, Mr John Hunter and Sir Joseph Banks were elected "Honorary and Corresponding Members" of the College. Baker was physician to George III; Hunter, the great comparative anatomist and surgeon, was head of the surgical profession; Banks, explorer and patron of science, was President of the Royal Society. The prestige of this patronage was matched only by the subscribing support of the Prince of Wales and the Duke of York.

At an important meeting in April 1791, the Duke of Northumberland agreed to be president of the College. There were eight vice-presidents, of the highest social standing. Eighteen other gentlemen of substance were elected directors, and another fifteen were nominated honorary and corresponding members because of their knowledge of the veterinary art. These latter were continental acquaintances of St Bel, or heads of various veterinary schools in Europe; there was, of course, no British veterinarian to join such company. The number of patrons of the school grew rapidly — notable, wealthy and influential people. Granville Penn was delighted by so much enthusiasm.

In discussing a site for the school, St Bel pointed out at a meeting in September 1791 that "animals are more frequently attacked by epizootic, endemic and contagious diseases than the human species because we are protected from these casualties by our Houses, Clothing and manner of living and in short by all the precautions that reason dictates, whilst animals are deprived of all these resources and are constantly exposed to damages which we avoid by the above mentioned precautions, besides their food and drink is constantly the same which often is the cause of a fermentation in their blood which generally terminates in stubborn and fatal diseases." He stressed the need to build the school away from "marshy and low ground," because it "exhales very unwholesome and putrid vapours."

Even allowing for the translator-cum-transcriber's difficulty in keeping up with St Bel's quick-fire French (for he spoke little English), there is no mistaking his perpetuation of the age-old belief in evil humours and unwholesome miasmata as important causes of disease. On the same occasion, St Bel made an assessment of the relative respectability of veterinary and human medicine. He insisted that medical students should not be allowed to attend his lectures, "becasue it might give a disgust to the residing pupils from their application to the veterinary medicine and many of them would change their mind and apply themselves to the anatomy of the human body, thinking that it would be more honorable for them to cure the human species than animals."

A site for the London school was found near St Pancras church, on land belonging to Lord Camden. A house was available for St Bel, and a temporary building was erected close by so that teaching could start without delay.

When lectures began on 4th January 1792, there were four resident pupils, all sponsored by subscribers to the College. By the end of the year the number had increased to fourteen, with additional non-resident pupils. Rules for resident pupils were strict. All had to attend a place of worship; London was out-of-bounds; entry and exit were to be by the gates, not over the walls; the Professor's lectures were strictly private. And so on. At a meeting of the governing Council on 9th August 1792, the porter was instructed "not to suffer under any pretence whatever either drinking or gaming in his Lodge." At this meeting detailed regulations were drawn up for porters, smiths, the Secretary, and the Professor. Everyone must understand that this was a serious venture, and that high moral and educational standards were necessary for those pursuing the Veterinary Art.

The course of instruction was planned to last three years, with morning and afternoon classes for most of the year. Emphasis, inevitably, was on the horse, but study of "epoizootic diseases of farm animals" was specifically part of the curriculum. Pupils came from all over England. Some in their young teens, others in maturing twenties. In general, they had a good educational background, and some had had medical training. The social position of supporters of the school was reflected in these earliest pupils.

A programme of permanent building was started in 1792, but this led to financial embarrassment, for costs exceeded the income from pupils' fees and support subscriptions. A loan of £2,000 was obtained early in 1793, an inopportune financial moment with the country shaken by the guillotined Louis XVI and France's declaration of war against England.

More serious than strained finances, however, was the discovery that a number of non-resident students had defected and set up in practice, declaring that they had been trained at the London veterinary school. This necessitated widespread newspaper advertising that "no person has yet quitted the College as qualified to practise Farriery," and that a Certificate would be granted only after "a strict Publick examination."

But neither unsatisfactory finance nor unqualified practice was of moment by comparison with the calamity of August 1793. St Bel died in the middle of that month, after a brief illness. Because to a great extent St Bel *was* the school, the school nearly died with him. By good fortune, however, the pupils, behaving with great responsibility, managed to maintain the hospital, and John Hunter bridged the educational gap until another Professor could be found by arranging for medical colleagues to take the veterinary men into their classes.

The school was without a Professor for seven months. The search for a replacement for St Bel was delegated to a group of medical subscribers to the school who, in October 1792, had formed themselves into a "Medical Experimental Committee," with the objective of making studies in comparative medicine. The members of this Committee were Sir George Baker, Sir William Fordyce, Doctor Crawford, Doctor Scott, Mr Hunter, Mr Cline and Mr Houlston. It was fortuitous — and historically significant — that these men were asked to undertake this executive task.

The field of candidates for the Professorship was restricted in the extreme. The only formally trained British veterinarian at the time was William Moorcroft, an able young man who had been encouraged by John Hunter to spend a year at the French veterinary school in Lyons, and who, early in 1792, had set up practice in London. Now, at Hunter's suggestion, an attempt was made to interest him in the London school. But Moorcroft had no wish to abandon his practice, although he did agree to help out until a permanent appointment was made. Only one application for the post was received. This was from Edward Coleman, a human surgeon, twenty-eight years old, also known to Hunter, and, more intimately, to another member of the Committee, Henry Cline, in whose house Coleman had lived while studying at medical school in London. In the event, the dual appointment was made in February 1794 of Moorcroft and Coleman. Moorcroft resigned, however, after a few weeks, leaving Coleman undisputed leader of an emerging profession. This appointment completely altered the outlook of the London veterinary school. It was of a medical man by medical men. Could St Bel's veterinary Plan, so painstakingly prepared, still prosper?

The answer was that no Professor who was not a veterinarian could carry out the Plan. The medical outlook, then as now, is different from the veterinary. It may seem that because disease is so similar in man and animals, medical and veterinary thinking must be essentially the same. It is not so. In many ways the professions are poles apart — in psychology, for example, and economics. Animals never imagine they are ill. By contrast, psychosomatic illness in man is commonplace. No medical man can consider euthanasia an alternative to pain and misery. A physically handicapped human being can live happily in mind and spirit, but a sickly animal is discarded by its tribe. From earliest times it has been said that the medical is superior to the veterinary art, for man is assumed to be nobler than the brute. But like can only be compared with like, and the medical and veterinary arts are different.

It is conceivable that if John Hunter's guidance had been available to the young Coleman, the school might have continued to develop in a veterinary fashion, but Hunter died in October 1793 and his feeling and sympathy for animals died with him.

Edward Coleman is one of a small number of people who have claimed some attention from the even smaller number of people who have written about British veterinary history. Coleman has not been readily assessed. Some have found nothing in his favour, and much for which to damn him in perpetuity. Others have taken a more liberal view of faults and have offered modest praise. A few have opined that, although tedious, his behaviour during a reign of forty-five years over the London school was no more reprehensible than that of other mediocrities vouchsafed autocracy by circumstance.

The significance of Coleman's friendship with Astley Cooper, however, is acknowledged by all. Cooper — later Sir Astley Cooper, premier surgeon of his day — has survived in biography as a considerable figure. He described Coleman as having "an acute and active mind." The two were students together in surgeon Henry Cline's house in London. They attended John Hunter's lectures; they talked and argued, as young men will, and theirs was friendship for a lifetime. Through Cooper, Coleman was constantly in touch with medical men. He learned a little about the ills of horses, but was wont to say that animals were simpler than people and their diseases were simpler, too.

Coleman made a special study of horse-shoes and shoeing. The extent of his expertise has been recorded by Bransby Blake Cooper in a biography (dated 1843) of his uncle Sir Astley Cooper: "I remember about fifteen years ago, having purchased a fine black horse, I rode him up immediately to my friend Coleman, and asked him his opinion of my purchase. He examined him carefully, extolled his points, flattered me on my judgement, but said, 'He has a slight tendency to contraction of his heels. Go to our forge directly, have my shoes put on him, and you will prevent the mischief to which he seems obnoxious.' Having done as he recommended, I mounted the horse immediately afterwards, and no cat in pattens could go more lame. I dared not, however, ride him back to the college to have his shoes taken off, but took him to Turner's, in Regent Street, where common shoes were again put on, and I never knew him go a yard unsound afterwards."

Lest it be considered unfair to Coleman's "acute and active mind" to quote what might be an isolated instance of veterinary ineptitude, it is proper to record something of his knowledge of other diseases. After all, lameness in horses can still puzzle experts. Coleman's knowledge of animal disease was restricted to horses, however, for he was unassailable in a lifelong opinion that diseases of other animals were unworthy of veterinary notice.

In 1796, after two years as head of the London school, he published: "Instructions for the use of Farriers attached to the British Cavalry and the Honourable Board of Ordnance." By now he had the confidence of the school's Governors, who liked his urbane manner and administrative competence. He was affable with the students, and lectured in expansive fashion. It was not held against him that he had made no attempt to implement St Bel's Plan for a three-year course on the anatomy, physiology and diseases of all domesticated animals.

It is unnecessary to quote in detail Coleman's booklet of instructions to Army farriers. His guidance on the disease called 'staggers' will suffice: "*Symptoms*. When this disease first makes its appearance, the animal is very much disposed to sleep, and while standing his head nearly approaches the ground; this is commonly called sleeping staggers. If this complaint is not soon removed, it becomes more violent, and the horse continually attempts to run round, and is in a state of high delirium; this is called mad staggers, but is the same disease in *kind*, differing only in degree. *Treatment*. The horse should lose at least four quarts of blood, and repeated every four hours during the first twelve, if the symptoms be not relieved. The top of the head should be blistered (the hair being first cut close), one ounce and half of the laxative powder . . . should be given immediately, or even two ounces if the horse be large. The hair should be cut off from the hoof to the fetlock joints, and boiling water poured on the part; this should be repeated twice in the day. Clysters of warm water and salt should be given every two hours (one pound of salt to five quarts of water). If the horse do not purge in thirty-six hours after the first powder has been given, repeat the dose, as before. Two rowels should be placed under his belly."

In explanation: a clyster was an enema, and a rowel was a piece of leather about an inch in diameter with a hole in the centre, forced under the skin through an incision, to cause suppuration and drainage for evil humours.

It may reasonably be inferred from this ghastly little book that Edward Coleman was not an ideal mentor for young men who aspired to work with animals. He betrays, too, an insensitivity almost beyond belief.

This insensitivity stood him in good personal stead, however, when applied to other matters. In 1796 he agreed to a war-emergency shortening of the veterinary course, so that every cavalry regiment might quickly have a veterinary surgeon. When this immediate require-ment for veterinary surgeons had been met, he saw no reason to revert to the longer course. After all, the shorter the course, the more students could be processed, and the greater the number of students the greater his income from their fees. So attendance at the school for only a few months became the rule, with no educational requirement restricting entry. The veterinary course became popular with all sorts of folk, from those who could both read and write to those who could scarcely do either. The examination was, of course, entirely verbal. It was con-ducted by a Board exclusively of medical men (of great eminence, be it said, in their own sphere), with Astley Cooper in the chair. Coleman indicated to this Board the students who were worthy of a certificate of competence in the Veterinary Art.

Insensitivity was helpful, too, when Coleman was appointed in 1796 (at his own suggestion) veterinary adviser to the Army. Clinical ignorance was no deterrent to drawing the stipend of ten shillings per day (doubled on inspection days), and one shilling and threepence per mile travelling allowance, a useful addition to professorial earnings. His fees as Army adviser were not begrudged however, for it is in this capacity that he has acquired approbation from those who have not consigned him totally to perdition. His advice to exchange the traditional sealed and stifling stable for a system open to the airs of heaven, was followed by an almost magical improvement in the health of Army horses. This success brought great renown, and his advice on veterinary matters — even topical application, twice daily, of boiling water — was above reproach. What was not mentioned (even if it were known) was that Coleman's system of stable husbandry had been described in detail by James Clark, Royal Farrier in Scotland, in 1788. But who would be so mean as to wonder if Coleman's fresh-air stables really *did* emanate from his "acute and active mind?" After all, James Clark was a Scotsman. Probably uncouth, to boot.

Much less is known about the day-by-day affairs of the London veteri-nary school during the first quarter of the nineteenth century than in any other period of its history. There are three reasons. First, there was no journal interested to report veterinary matters. Secondly, Coleman governed secretly. Thirdly, the institution was intellectually moribund. Students arrived, stayed for a few months, then went on their way, rejoic-ing in a crisp certificate of competency in the Veterinary Art.

The Governors, and the Examining Board led by Astley Cooper, were well satisfied with Edward Coleman. Few problems interrupted the cosiness of the Club that ruled the school. The financial difficulties of the early St Bel days had been eliminated by a Government grant in 1795 of £1,500, stimulated by the need for veterinary surgeons for the French war. This grant was repeated annually until 1813. Coleman himself had no financial worries. Students' fees, Army consultancies, and adroit manipulation of various perquisites raised his income to an estimated £3,500 annually by the 1820's (equivalent in 1980 to £70,000 free of tax).

A Demonstrator of Anatomy, William Sewell, was appointed to help Coleman in 1799, immediately after receiving his diploma from the school. A grey man, a Quaker, who seldom left the precincts of the school, he was content to be Coleman's shadow and factotum. Once in Coleman's lifetime, in 1815, Sewell sallied forth into the world, to visit Continental veterinary schools. The banality of his report on that expedition has to be read to be believed. He did, however, discover the central canal of the spinal cord. Characteristically, he did not himself publicise his discovery (on which many another might have dined for a lifetime), but his letter to the Royal Society was published in the *Philosophical Transactions* for 1809.

Late in life, Coleman was elected a Fellow of the Royal Society. After forty years, merit was suddenly recognised in observations on suspended animation he had made (while studying medicine) by asphyxiating large numbers of dogs. This reason for election to the Society is so unconvincing that it seems but an excuse to join Sir Astley Cooper and other cronies in the Citadel, by way of its social postern. Coleman's Fellowship of the Royal Society has been cited as the first election of a member of the veterinary profession to that Society. The claim is untenable, however, because he was not a veterinary surgeon, by inclination or training, and he died before the veterinary profession was born.

Coleman's attitude was paternal towards his students. As he grew older he referred to "my children" but he seems to have overlooked the perception of childhood. Not a few of his children who had entered the London veterinary school with a wish to study and to live with animals, were soon aware of how little it had to offer. Disappointment bred dissatisfaction, then mild complaint.

In 1824 Joseph Goodwin, veterinary surgeon to George IV, asked at the annual meeting of subscribers to the school that veterinary surgeons be included in the Examining Board. His motion was haughtily dismissed by the Governors as not in the interests of the pupils.

Goodwin, himself medically trained (a contemporary of Coleman and Cooper at Guy's Hospital), deeply resented this snub, and from that moment pioneered a movement to reform the school. He teamed up with

Army veterinary surgeon Frederick Clifford Cherry, another tough character, a veteran of Waterloo, and seized every opportunity to criticise the existing regime and to press for improvements. By March 1827 these two had succeeded in persuading an unwilling Coleman to sign a document setting out such revolutionary changes as veterinary examiners, instruction on diseases of dogs and farm animals, experimental measurement of the effects of medicines, and payment for the extra expenditure involved by deduction of five guineas from the fee paid to Coleman by each pupil.

Coleman did nothing to implement the document. As always, he had full support from the ruling clique.

It was now plain not only to Goodwin and Cherry but also to the many who supported them, that only a frontal attack could force reforms upon the school.

The attack was launched in 1828.

CHAPTER 2

Criticism of the school — Hopes for a professional charter

On 1st January 1828, broadsides were fired at Edward Coleman and the London veterinary school from cannon embedded in the pages of the first two veterinary periodicals to be published in Britain. It was coincidental that the first number of each journal appeared on the same day, for neither editor knew for certain of the existence of the other. That each should have had the purpose of publicising inadequacies of the London school, however, emphasises a generalised rise in the temperature of simmering criticism.

These journals, both monthlies, were *The Farrier and Naturalist* (later renamed *The Hippiatrist*), and *The Veterinarian*. Reform of the London school was a major objective for each, but their styles could scarcely have been more disparate.

The Farrier and Naturalist was published anonymously for three years. It concentrated on attacking Coleman personally. Its criticism was blunt and repetitive: "We do not hesitate to assert that the Veterinary College is one of the most rotten public establishments in England: but . . . we have it in our power to considerably reduce the mass of corruption by which . . . the profession is degraded."

It is believed that the senior editor of this journal was Bracy Clark, who disliked Coleman from the day the Professor was appointed to lead the London school, a few months before Clark obtained his veterinary diploma. Clark was well educated before becoming one of the school's first pupils, under St Bel, and on graduating he established a lucrative practice in the City of London. He was a considerable naturalist, a linguist, a writer, and an inventor of items as diverse as fireworks and a shaving-box for travellers. He was also bad-tempered and unforgiving. Other Coleman-haters contributed to *The Farrier and Naturalist*, and the invective was enthusiastically maintained.

By contrast, *The Veterinarian* was envisaged by its founder and first editor, William Percivall, as a journal for the whole profession, through which there would be communication on the widest range of subjects. Criticism of the London school was a high priority, certainly, but it had to be informed and constructive, and must be leavened by clinical and scientific articles, abstracts from foreign journals, news items and editorials. It was a new veterinary venture, and right well did it succeed. The standard of production was high, and the standard of writing higher still.

William Percivall was thirty-six years old when the first number of *The Veterinarian* was published. He received his veterinary diploma from the London school in 1811, was veterinary surgeon to the Ordnance in the Peninsular war, qualified as a human surgeon in 1819, and wrote extensively on the anatomy and diseases of the horse. In launching *The Veterinarian* he had great support from his father John Percivall, who, for thirty years, was veterinary surgeon to the Ordnance at Woolwich. Indeed, the objectives of this new journal were formulated by father and son, and special consideration was given to the manner in which criticism of the London school was to be handled. The point here was that John Percivall had been appointed to Woolwich on Coleman's recommendation, and the two had worked closely together. Although John Percivall disagreed with Coleman's methods, he was not prepared to condone spiteful criticism. He said: "Pursue the course you have worked out . . . it is worthy of *The Veterinarian* and of you. Attack, expose the measures . . . but spare the man . . . your work belongs to the profession, and dare ever to shew that you are in the slightest degree influenced by malignity or revenge, and I will disown the *The Veterinarian* and you."

William Percivall had expected *The Veterinarian* to take off with a bang. Instead, there was an almost inaudible pop. He had anticipated that his colleagues would submit articles and news items, so that his pages would readily be filled. But the idea of professional communication through public writing was so novel among veterinary surgeons, that there was almost a year's delay before the initial trickle of material became a steady flow. In the meantime a disillusioned Percivall had to write a great part of the first twelve numbers. He had a staunch comrade, however, in William Youatt who joined him as an editor in the early days of the venture. Born in 1776, Youatt had originally studied for the Nonconformist ministry, but when well into his thirties he was drawn into the veterinary world by a feeling for animals, and became a pupil of Delabere Blaine who had a large practice in London. Blaine persuaded him to attend the veterinary school, but Coleman vented on Youatt a dislike for Blaine, to the extent that after a few months Youatt left the school without a diploma. His maturity, however, and deep concern for animals were appreciated by Blaine, who took him into partnership. Youatt spread his interest over all animal species (most unusual at the time), and eventually delivered annually a well patronised course of lectures on their diseases. He wrote well and was an ideal person to join Percivall on *The Veterinarian*.

The influence of *The Veterinarian* on the development of the British veterinary profession cannot be exaggerated, and it is thrice fortunate that it was produced by men of the ability and integrity of William Percivall and William Youatt. It brought a scattered profession together, and made possible the reforms so urgently needed.

Pressure of a different character was also brought to bear on the London school in the 1820s. A rival veterinary school was established by William Dick in Edinburgh. London and Edinburgh were too far apart by stage-coach or pack-horse for rivalry in the sense of one school stealing pupils from the other, but the fact of a second school invited comparison with the first. Dick, a farrier's son, born in Edinburgh, had undertaken the journey to London in 1817 to find out for himself the truth in rumours of a veterinary school. His diploma from the London school was dated 27th January 1818, granted after some three months' tuition. Back in Edinburgh, the anatomist Dr Barclay encouraged him to widen his veterinary knowledge by reading and practice at his father's forge. With considerable tenacity over the next few years he continued this self-education, and gave occasional lectures. In 1823, again with Barclay's backing, he obtained the patronage of the Highland and Agricultural Society for a course of veterinary lectures, the first of which was given on 24th November 1823 at the Calton Convening Rooms. The lectures were a success, and encouraged Dick to found the Edinburgh veterinary school, for which funds — hard earned — came from his practice. The school prospered. The Highland and Agricultural Society willingly continued its patronage, and issued, on behalf of the school, certificates of veterinary competence to pupils approved by an examining board of medical and veterinary men.

The extent to which the London veterinary school of the 1820's was an entrenched monopoly in England, may be gauged from the tale of the attempt in 1829 to achieve two small modifications in its administration. First, to have veterinary surgeons represented on the Examining Board, and secondly to allow veterinary surgeons to be subscribers to the school. With regard to the latter, it is well-nigh incredible that of all classes of society — high, low and medium — veterinary surgeons alone were excluded from subscribing to the school. The reason given by the

Governors was that veterinary surgeons "might learn some of the secrets of the College" thus "becoming more skilful and successful", with the result that they "might interfere with the interests and lessen the profits of the College."

In order to discuss these points informally with Coleman, a dinner was arranged at the Freemasons' Tavern in London on 22nd April 1829, with the Professor in the chair. In an atmosphere of superficial cordiality, "nearly forty practitioners" enjoyed an excellent meal, and "after the cloth was withdrawn", drank to "The King," "The Duke of Clarence, President of the Veterinary College," "The Royal Family," and "The Duke of Wellington."

William Youatt then proposed "The Royal Veterinary College."

He was ever so polite, but ever so firm, ending his speech by saying: "The time, sir, is not far distant when this institute will fulfil the admirable purposes of its excellent founders — will be more identified with the agricultural interests of the country — no longer our disgrace, but our pride and our boast; — a national institution, wisely planned, well conducted and eminently useful."

Coleman (who detested Youatt) replied effusively. He thanked the company "for the honour you have done the institution, and for the honour you have done me in proposing this toast; as well as for the manner in which you have received and drunk it." With practised circumlocution, he averred that the two points at issue were at all times in his consciousness, and that it was for the assembled company to make propositions that he would be pleased to put to the Governors.

A brief discussion was adjourned, by common consent, to another occasion "when the pleasures of the bottle might not seduce us from graver considerations."

A few days later, a widely advertised meeting, that lasted from seven o'clock until after midnight, eventually agreed that memorials should be presented to the Examining Board of the London school, and to its Governors.

These memorials were restrained and factual documents, and it seemed that they could not be other than favourably received.

Less than a month later they were turned down, with polite contempt, and readers of *The Veterinarian* for 1st June 1829 shared their editor's anger and frustration.

Yet another meeting was summoned by public advertisement for 8th July 1829. Coleman appeared after the meeting had started. He was offered the chair, but declined, declaring: "I came for a specific purpose — to explain the result of the honour conferred upon me by presenting the memorials, and to answer any questions . . . Having discharged this duty . . . I shall retire, that the matter may be discussed without restraint."

He left the meeting a short time later, and Frederick Cherry commented: "Not a single syllable of what Mr Coleman has now stated applied to the business of the present meeting."

What could be done? From the debate that followed, two points of view emerged. One advised continued co-operation with Coleman and the Governors, in the hope that time might bring the desired improvements. The other argued that the school should be abandoned, and that an entirely separate examining committee of veterinary surgeons should be created, to issue certificates of strictly veterinary competence to anyone prepared to face and satisfy the committee. Between these extremes there was ample room for discussion. Discussion there certainly was; argument, too, accusation and acrimony, with comments such as: ". . . puerile, ridiculous and involved in absurdity."

But a new idea suddenly appeared. James Child said: ". . . the College diploma is ridiculed . . . why is this? Because the College is a mere private institution, and not a chartered body . . .   Nothing can be done effectually until, as a body, we apply for a charter."

Wise, prophetic words, but lost in the clamour and confusion.

Those in favour of a separate veterinary examining committee believed that their proposition had been accepted. Midnight again caused adjournment. The final act was played out two weeks later. It was a shambles. The chair was taken without authority by "Mr Trowse (whose name does not appear in the list of veterinary surgeons)." The meeting had been infiltrated by supporters of the *status quo*. By whom recruited? There was everything short of fisticuffs. Those who had wished to create a veterinary committee retired in disgust. The meeting was adjourned *sine die*. William Youatt, champion of moderation and reasoned action, reporting for *The Veterinarian*, was appalled. Finally, referring to the malcontents' refusal to pay for the room, he recorded: ". . . the evening concluded leaving it in the power of the landlord to say that representatives of the body of veterinary surgeons had assembled in his house and bilked him of his just demand for the use of the room."

Sir Astley Cooper, Edward Coleman, the Governors of the London veterinary school — and the bully boys — had won.

Referring to these meetings in *The Veterinarian* some years later, Youatt wrote: "They were fearful and disgraceful times."

Little wonder that those who dreamed in 1829 of a worthwhile veterinary profession had to sleep awhile and dream again.

There is a post-script to this episode. A letter dated 10th June 1830 from Coleman to Thomas Walton Mayer, sixteen years old, veterinary-surgeon-to-be, son of Thomas Mayer, respected veterinary surgeon of Newcastle-under-Lyme:-

"My dear Sir,
    Many thanks for your valuable cheese which is excellent — and for the kind interest you have taken in my behalf against a few Individuals who have exerted their utmost to drive me from my Chair, and one of them stated he would never cease to exert himself to obtain that object. They want the loaves and fishes and try hard to get rid of Mr Sewell and myself, but they could not agree as to the division of the spoil. My best wishes for your health and happiness and believe me to be
Yours truly obliged,
Edw Coleman
My compliments to your Father and family

Clearly, Edward Coleman (now sixty-five years old) had no intention of changing his ways nor of resigning his post.

At that time, however, all was not veterinary disgrace, in spite of Edward Coleman and his school. Here and there, there were veterinarians of ability and integrity. One such was John Field, born in 1768, son and grandson of farriers, who, in 1794, joined William Moorcroft in practice in London's Oxford Street. An obituary notice by Youatt in *The Veterinarian* of 1833 recalls this man. In particular, he was skilled "in that portion of a veterinary surgeon's duty which consists in the examination of horses for purchase or sale," when "the discrimination and tact of the surgeon are temporarily bought as a defence against . . . the imposition of the seller." Field was angered by the many and varied tricks used to hide faults, "and to no man are we so much indebted for the discontinuance of many an infamous fraud. The public . . . approved of his system . . . he scrupled not to point out the faults of the horses of his best friends."

This high standard in the examination of horses set by John Field, and maintained by others through the nineteenth century, has been immortalised in the verb 'to vet.'

Change in the affairs of men is usually from without as well as from within. So it was with the veterinary world. Advances in education and status that were out of the question in 1829, lost their impossibility during the decade that followed. It was a period of profound social change. The industrial revolution gathering momentum. Railways and better roads, and movement of people. The Reform Bill and weakening of aristocratic monopoly. Improvement in agriculture. Expansion in trade. Within the profession there was an increasing corporate sense, built round *The Veterinarian*. Month after month that journal spread news, comment and technical information across the land. Dick of Edinburgh and Karkeek of Truro joined Percivall and Youatt on the editorial board in 1833, so that it could truthfully be said that there was a unifying influence from John o' Groat's house to Land's End. Foundation of the English Agricultural Society (later the Royal Agricultural Society) in 1838, brought recognition that success in "management, in health and disease, of our cattle and sheep . . . would be of inestimable advantage to the British farmer." Youatt, an early member of the Society and friend of its Secretary, persuaded the Society to include encouragement of veterinary education among its stated objectives.

Above all, within the profession, Edward Coleman died in 1839. No doubt he was mourned by friends, but his demise gave new hope of advancement to the profession he had obstructed for so long.

The Veterinarian's sigh of relief when Coleman died is patent in Youatt's editorial appraisal of the "gentleman" who "departed this life on the evening of Sunday the 14th July." This memoir begins with the story of the London school briefly told; the characteristically generous comment on Coleman is: "Let him pass!" He had his good points as well as his bad." Then Youatt turns with enthusiasm to the future. He sketches a plan for the school, with emphasis on instruction in anatomy, physiology and pathology of all the domesticated animals. He urges that the course be lengthened to two years, for all who have not been apprenticed to a veterinary surgeon. Youatt accurately assessed the changes that were required, because the eventual improvements in the school's curriculum were closely similar to these suggestions.

William Sewell, Coleman's sycophant and shadow for over forty years, was appointed Professor. It could scarcely have been otherwise, because no one else had even remotely similar experience. Radical change, therefore, was still out of the question. The most that could be prayed for was that, with Coleman out of the way, Sewell would find sufficient personality of his own to co-operate in plans to modify the *status quo*. Charles Spooner became Assistant Professor. Spooner had established a private school in veterinary anatomy in 1834, and four years later became a lecturer at the London school. Chemistry and materia medica were in the benevolent hands of William John Thomas Morton, who had joined the school in 1822 as a clerk and dispenser. The most important advance, however, came slightly later with the appointment in 1842 to the new post of Professor of Cattle Pathology of James Beart Simonds, one of only a handful of veterinary surgeons at that time with real experience of disease in farm animals. This crucial professorship was financed through the generosity of the Royal Agricultural Society.

It has been noted that at a meeting in 1829 James Child declared that professional recognition could only be by charter, but his words were lost in the general confusion. A year later the same proposition was ably expounded in a letter to *The Veterinarian* by W. Simpson, a practitioner in Lancaster. In 1834 *The Veterinarian* took up and pressed the idea, and from that time it became increasingly clear that the only possibility of advance lay along the road to legal recognition of professional status.

As soon as the Coleman obstruction had been removed, a first step was taken by Thomas Mayer and Thomas Walton Mayer, father and son practitioners in Newcastle-under-Lyme. The Mayers had been friendly with Coleman, while not sharing his professional views, and it was from Thomas Walton Mayer that Coleman had received the welcomed cheese. Now they sent to every veterinary surgeon in the Kingdom, the draft of a memorial addressed to the Governors of the London veterinary school, politely seeking co-operation in improving the course of instruction and in establishing relations between the school and the agricultural community. Practitioners were asked to support this memorial. Mayer junior preserved the large number of replies received, and, late in life, presented them to the Royal College of Veterinary Surgeons. They vividly express goodwill and support from colleagues everywhere.

In response to this favourable reaction, the Mayers announced in *The Veterinarian* for May 1840: "We will not conceal that we have ulterior views. When we have made the education of the veterinary surgeon that which it ought to be . . . we shall have a right to think of, and to supplicate from the powers that be, 'a Charter of Incorporation', to protect us from illiterate and uneducated men, and to afford us the same privileges and exemptions which other professional bodies possess." Commenting editorially on the Mayer initiative, Youatt wrote: "The name of Mayer will be added to the list of those who have done our profession service, and our children's children will have to thank them."

On 10th June 1840 an eight-man deputation, led by Thomas Turner, was courteously received by the Governors of the London veterinary school. The memorial was discussed, and a case — ably presented by Mayer junior — was made for the Governors to support application for a charter. It was pointed out by the Governors, however, that although a charter might create a profession in name, legal protection could only be by Act of Parliament. The Governors professed to be impressed by arguments presented on behalf of a majority of veterinary surgeons in the country. Their considered reply to the memorial would be given in due course.

That reply, dated 3rd July 1840 and addressed to "Messers Mayer and Son", stated that the Governors "do not see the immediate necessity for applying to the Crown for a Royal Charter to be granted to this Institution; but that every facility would be given to the veterinary surgeons for procuring an Act of Parliament to prevent certain grievances complained of by the Memorial, which could not be relieved by a charter."

In other words, the ball was lobbed back into the Mayers' court.

Thomas Walton Mayer accepted the challenge, and set about a task later described by an admiring colleague as "little short of Herculean."

He organised a meeting of veterinary surgeons who had signed the memorial to the Governors of the London school, at which it was decided to petition the Privy Council for a Royal Charter "conferring upon the graduates of the Royal Veterinary College and the College of Edinburgh the title of the Royal College of Veterinary Surgeons, upon the same plan and constitution as the present Royal College of Surgeons." He became Secretary of a Standing Committee of veterinary surgeons dedicated to reaching this objective. His was the responsibility for arranging meetings, presenting petitions, organising deputations, collecting subscriptions, urging, pleading, chivvying, prodding. And all this, be it recalled, without telegraph, telephone, typewriter, carbon paper or internal combustion engine. To say nothing of out-of-pocket expenses.

It is not surprising that months became years before the charter application — checked, re-checked, pruned and polished — at last was ready for dispatch.

As a pleasant change from earlier argument and obstruction, progress was steady towards a veterinary charter from 1840 onwards. There was significant support in both Houses of Parliament, and William Dick, founder, owner and Professor of the Edinburgh school, signified approval in 1841. In April 1842 a deputation to the Home Secretary, Sir James Graham, received good advice and guarded encouragement. In February 1843 the co-operation was obtained of the London school professors William Sewell and Charles Spooner, and a month later the application was submitted to the Home Office.

The Standing Committee of veterinary surgeons had ballotted for names to be attached to this precious document. Thomas Turner, William Joseph Goodwin, William Dick and Thomas Mayer senior had been chosen. In addition, as a gesture of courtesy to the London school, the names of the three professors William Sewell, Charles Spooner and

James Beart Simonds were added. Of these latter, Simonds had been a founder member of the Standing Committee and regular attender at its meetings, but Sewell and Spooner had contributed nothing but last-minute acquiescence.

April 1843 came and went, then May, and June . . . and Christmas. There was no word from the Privy Council office, no sign.

It was hard to wait so long with bated breath.

CHAPTER 3

The charter achieved in 1844

Lest it be inferred that the major veterinary activity in the early 1840's was political, it must be emphasised that active attempts to improve professional education and status (as distinct from widespread complaint about the veterinary lot) were limited to a handful of men who — with the notable exception of the Mayers — lived in or near London. For the remainder of the profession (an undetermined number at the time, but probably several hundreds) politics were something to be discussed by others in *The Veterinarian*. The struggle for existence against double their number of unqualified horse-doctors and cow-leeches left little time for political activity. There were no veterinary associations in rural areas where colleagues could meet, and the professional isolation of many country practitioners was absolute.

In these circumstances, the importance of *The Veterinarian* in broadcasting technical information was enormous. Thus, in the September number for 1839, Mr Hill, V.S. of Islington Green, warned the profession of an alarming new disease among cows in dairies close to London. The most obvious clinical signs were "inflammation and vesication" of "the membrane of the whole of the mouth," and "a continual catching up and shaking of one or the other of the hind-legs." Very soon other practitioners encountered this disease, referred to at first as "the vesicular epizootic," or "malignant epidemic murrain," then as "mouth-and-foot disease," and finally as foot-and-mouth disease. The origin of the disease was a matter for conjecture, but majority opinion favoured spontaneous generation initiated by abnormal atmospheric conditions; too much rain, or too little; too much sunshine, or not enough; too much heat, too much cold. Anything, in fact, that did not fit with the expected weather for the time of year. Such a theory was thoroughly satisfactory, because no one could prove it wrong.

Only in delayed retrospect was it noticed that the first appearance in

Britain of foot-and-mouth disease coincided with the political decision to establish free trade with countries across the seas. The Free Trade doctrine covered free trade in animals, but it was not realised that it also included free trade in their diseases.

Apprehensive about the new disease, the Royal Agricultural Society turned for advice to the London veterinary school. Coleman had recently died, but Sewell confidently described treatment. *Viz*: copper sulphate for sore mouths and feet; setons in the throat or dewlap (a seton being a thick string or tape drawn by needle through a fistful of skin and sub-cutaneous flesh, and left to suppurate); blisters and bleeding; calomel if there appeared to be dysfunction of the liver; soda and ginger if the bowels were disturbed; opium and fomentations if there was evidence of pain. In short, he had not a clue as to the origin, nature or course of the disease, and had neither the wit nor the honesty to say so. His advice spread the disease across the land. No wonder that in 1842 the Royal Agricultural Society agreed to subsidise a professorship in Cattle Pathology at the London school.

James Beart Simonds, first Professor of Cattle Pathology, saw foot-and-mouth disease in his practice at Twickenham in 1839, and carried out perhaps the earliest transmission experiment with the disease in Britain. He rubbed hay over the mouth of an affected cow, then fed the hay to a healthy cow. The disease appeared in the second animal. He knew, therefore, that the disease could spread by contact between affected and healthy animals, but he believed that it had developed orig-inally by spontaneous generation. The belief — general at the time — that the disease had not been imported into Britain but had arisen spontaneously, was conditioned by the fact that free trade in live animals had not properly begun when the disease suddenly appeared in widely separated localities. What neither Simonds nor anyone else at the time could know, was that hides and other animal products already being imported from the Continent, could readily carry the infection of foot-and-mouth disease. This hidden and unsuspected passive transfer of infection from place to place, gave generations of respectability to the theory of spontaneous origin of infectious diseases.

The Privy Council's reply to the charter petition was received eleven months after the application had been lodged. It was announced at a meeting of the Standing Committee of Veterinary Surgeons on 16th February 1844, Thomas Turner in the chair. Turner savoured the moment, holding his eight colleagues briefly in suspense: "Since the last meeting of the Committee I have . . . endeavoured . . . to obtain from Her Majesty's Government that Charter which we fondly hope will prove

. . . the salvation of the Veterinary body. It would be trespassing on your time . . . to enter into minute details . . . the obstacles that have been surmounted . . . the interviews that have taken place . . ."

After a few minutes he came to the point, with as momentous a statement as has ever been made by a veterinary chairman to a veterinary audience: "I am now able to congratulate you on our success and to announce that Her Majesty has been pleased to sign the warrants for our Charter."

It was a notable achievement, well summarised in a letter dated 25th February 1844 from William Dick of Edinburgh to Secretary Mayer:-

"My Dear Sir,
    I am glad to learn that you have succeeded in obtaining the Charter; I certainly did not expect it; circumstances; however, have been favourable. The present Ministers coming into power, and the agitation for the New Charter by the College of Surgeons, have aided much in enabling us to obtain what at first appeared to me very unlikely. I hope you will be as successful in obtaining from Parliament those privileges to which, as an incorporated body, we are entitled.
    I have received your circular and would have sent you a remittance, but am anxious to know what is my share, which, although I have not yet sent any portion of, I have held myself responsible, and shall be glad to hear from you as to the amount.
                                    W. Dick"

It was unnecessary to trouble Dick for a donation, for the £700 required to pay the immediate cost of the Charter had already been raised. As soon as the success of the application was announced by Chairman Turner, the delighted members of the Standing Committee agreed to lend the money to the "body corporate" at five per cent interest, in individual sums that ranged from £50 to £200. The remainder of the total Charter expenses — some £1,000 — was subscribed within six weeks in smaller sums sent from all over the country.

The reaction of *The Veterinarian* to the Charter was rapturous. The complete document was printed in twenty framed pages of bold type, beginning: "Victoria, by the Grace of God . . .' and ending: "Witness ourself at our Palace at Westminster, this eighth day of March, in the seventh year of our reign. By Writ of the Privy Council. Edmunds."

Thomas Turner was named as first President.

It may be noted that the Charter was regally signed some three weeks *after* President Turner had announced the Privy Council's decision to grant it. Clearly, last-minute obstruction from Queen Victoria was not anticipated.

The provisions of the Charter were of great moment. Unequivocally it created a new profession. This was to be composed of all persons holding the Certificate of the Veterinary College of London or the Veterinary College of Edinburgh, or any other duly authorised college in the future. All Members were to form one body, to be known as the Royal College of Veterinary Surgeons, which was a Corporation with power to buy, sell and act generally. It was directed that the Veterinary Art should henceforth be recognised as a profession, and that Members of the Corporation, solely and exclusively of all other persons, had the right to belong to the profession and to call themselves veterinary surgeons.

The Charter laid down rules for electing a President, Vice-Presidents, a Council and a Secretary, for calling and holding meetings, for engaging and removing servants. The defined responsibilities for examination of veterinary students were outstandingly important, and removed the power of examination from the schools. The Council was given power to make bye-laws to regulate examinations, to appoint examiners, to admit or reject students, and to determine examination and admission fees. No teacher at a veterinary school was permitted to be an examiner.

In conclusion, the property of the Royal College of Veterinary Surgeons was vested in the Corporation, and no sale or disposition was permissible without the College Council's approval.

This simple document was hailed as harbinger of a new veterinary era, and surely there would be no obstacle to obtaining the Act of Parliament essential to enforce its provisions.

The first general meeting of Members of the Royal College of Veterinary Surgeons (RCVS) was held in the afternoon of Friday 12th April 1844 at the Freemasons' Tavern, Great Queen Street, Lincoln's Inn Fields, with President Thomas Turner in the chair.

He opened the meeting with congratulations to one and all on acquisition of the Charter. The purpose of the meeting, he said, was to elect a Council of twenty-four, but first he would ask the Solicitor to read the Charter, so that its terms would be clearly understood.

Immediately after the Charter had been read, there was an inexplicable incident, enigmatically reported in *The Veterinarian*: "Professor Dick of Edinburgh, rose, and protested that, as several clauses had been introduced and others omitted in the Charter without his knowledge or consent, he should not be held as homologating the Charter by any part he might take in the business of the incorporation at its meetings on that occasion."

That was all. The report in *The Veterinarian* continued with details of the election of councillors, and Dick's expostulation received no further notice. This is an ominous blank in *The Veterinarian*'s usually extensive reporting. Something must very recently have upset Professor Dick, because on 25th February he had expressed goodwill in his letter to Mayer. The point is important, because Dick's co-operation was vital to the success of the RCVS.

It is difficult to diagnose the cause of annoyance. The Charter was so straightforward, was so long in the drafting, and was so widely discussed before it was sent to the Privy Council, that Dick must have been familiar with its major provisions. The most likely cause of irritation would be in the arrangements for examination of his students. Of this, however, no documentary evidence has been found, and, in any case, the examinations in Edinburgh were to be exactly as in London, apart from the composition of the Board of Examiners. Thomas Turner and Thomas Walton Mayer were not secretive people, and it would be out of character that they should have significantly modified the Charter without informing one of its most important signatories.

A possible explanation for Dick's abrupt antagonism may be compounded, first, of the fact that he was surprised when the Charter was granted (as stated in his letter to Mayer); secondly, that he and his school in Scotland were much less concerned to obtain a charter than the people in England, who were striving to throw off dominance by the London school; thirdly, that he had suddenly realised that the Charter would prevent him from examining his own students in his own school in his own way. Of these ingredients — recognising in Dick the pride of a Scotsman in his country and his people, and in his and their achievements — the third may be the most important.

After the William Dick intervention, twenty-four veterinary surgeons (including Dick) were elected to form the first ruling Council of the "body politic and corporate." In democratic fashion, they were grouped in sixes by date of graduation, from William Sewell 1799, to William Ernes 1839. These groups would retire annually in rotation, to be replaced annually by a newly-elected six, thus providing, after 1847, for all councillors to have four years in office.

A celebration dinner followed the Council election. At least eighteen toasts are identifiable, all drunk with enthusiasm. "Success to the Royal College of Veterinary Surgeons" was drunk "with all the honours and with vehement applause." Songs were contributed by the diners. Mr King junior, for example, rendered: " 'Oh, doth not a meeting like this make amends,' . . . with great taste and expression." Professor Dick made two good-humoured speeches, and towards the end of the evening "favoured the company with a song, 'John Anderson, my Jo.' "

A momentous occasion.

Three days later the Council met for the first time to elect six Vice-Presidents, a Treasurer (Francis King junior), and a Secretary (Edmund Gabriel). As examinations were imminent in both London and Edinburgh, a temporary Board of Examiners was appointed, and sub-committees were formed to decide on "a Seal and Diploma for the R.C.V.S.," to draw up bye-laws, and "to watch the progress of the Medical Reform Bill about to be introduced into Parliament, with the view of obtaining the privileges and exemptions petitioned for."

In short, the RCVS, truly born and now baptised, was on its way.

*　　*　　*

Although *The Veterinarian* made much of the Charter story, it did not forget its pledge to instruct as well as to inform its readers. It was especially anxious to report technical advances with practical potential. For example, the use of gaslight for singeing horses. It reported: "We are informed that it has recently occurred to the stud groom of a celebrated sportsman, whose stables are lit by gas, that the gaslight might be made subservient to the purpose of singeing his horses . . . he has had made a long flexible tube, screwed at one end into the gas-pipe, and to the other end has had fitted a burner similar in shape to that used for naphtha, only pierced with many small holes for the passage of the gas . . . he has had affixed to the burner a metallic horse-comb, standing in such situation and direction that, while he is carrying on his singeing operations, its teeth, by way of preparation to the burning, are furrowing and ruffling the hair . . . with his comb and burner together in one hand and a brush in the other, he rapidly performs his manipulations."

This inventive — not to say adventurous — groom found that he could "completely singe a horse in about four hours." The editors of *The Veterinarian* considered it a "marvel that it has not been thought of before," for the "soft lambent flame that gas produces" was so clearly preferable to "naphtha, or spirits of wine, or turpentine," and they recommended setting up "some place in or near town, whereto gentlemen might send their horses, and have them rid of their winter coats in a comparatively short space of time, at a cost something considerably less than is at present charged for the operation of tonsure."

*　　*　　*

High priority was given to devising a motto and arms for the RCVS, and within a few months of the signing of the Charter, "Chas. Geo. Young, *Garter*, J. Hawker, *Clarenceux*, and Frans. Martin, *Norroy*," had given their blessing to the motto and device proposed. The motto, *Vis unita fortior*, was not original either in a general or veterinary context. It had been the motto of William Harvey, renowned discoverer in 1628 of the circulation of the blood, and had been used (probably at the instigation of W.J.T. Morton, lecturer in chemistry at the London veterinary school) for the Veterinary Medical Association founded in 1836 as a discussion group for veterinary practitioners and students of the London school.

The official description of the Arms is: "Argent, a cross engrailed gules between a horse's head erased in the first quarter; an arrow in bend, entwined by and piercing a serpent in the second; a horseshoe in the third, all proper; and a bull's head, erased sable in the fourth." And of the Crest: "On a wreath of the colours, a centaur proper, holding a shield argent, charged with an aloe, also proper."

In less technical terms, the Arms are of a red cross with a wavy outside border, on a white shield, the four quarters of which show a horse's head, an arrow piercing a serpent, a horseshoe, and a bull's head. The heads of horse and bull are "erased," that is torn rather then severed from the body, and the arrow "in bend" in the second quarter runs diagonally from top right to bottom left (as viewed from the back of the shield). "Proper" signifies natural colouring. The horse and bull heads and the horseshoe indicate branches of the veterinary art. The healing arrow transfixes the serpent of disease. The white background is for purity of intent, and the red cross is self-sacrifice. The Crest is a centaur, perhaps Chiron, wisest of all the centaurs, skilled in medicine.

There is no doubt that at the moment of signing the RCVS Charter everything within the profession was sweetness and good humour. The past was past and the future glowed. This mood continued through the first meeting of Members, and even William Dick's remarks were critical of detail rather than hostile to a principle. The celebration dinner oozed bonhomie, and shortly afterwards, in an atmosphere approaching euphoria, sub-committees of the newly elected Council set about creating foundation bye-laws on which a practical and liberal administration might be built. As members of the Council, the London Professors Sewell, Spooner and Simonds were closely associated with these activities.

It was an astonished RCVS President Turner, therefore, who on 12th July 1844 (some eight weeks after the date of the Charter) received the following letter from the Home Office:-

"Sir,

I am directed by Secretary Sir James Graham to transmit to you the enclosed copies of two petitions, agreed to at a meeting of the Governors of and Subscribers to the Royal Veterinary College of London, holden on 1st instant.

Sir James Graham is desirous of receiving any answer or statement which the Council of the Royal College of Veterinary Surgeons may wish to make, especially with reference to the allegation that their Charter was obtained without the knowledge of the petitioners, and that there was an understanding between the parties that the proposed Charter, or instrument for that purpose, should be submitted to the Professor and Assistant Professors of the Royal Veterinary College London for their consideration, after all the provisions to be inserted had been set forth in it, and that it should contain nothing which could prove detrimental to the Royal Veterinary College of London — and that the full draft of such instrument was never submitted to them previously to its ultimate presentation, and that they were in ignorance of several provisions contained in it, which they now find will operate prejudicially to the said College.

I am, Sir,
Your obedient servant,
S.M. Phillips."

Turner's amazement turned to disbelief when he saw that the petitions were signed: "W. Sewell, On the part of the Governors." One of the documents was counter-signed: "Anglesey, Vice-President."

No more damning accusation could have been made against the RCVS. It was alleged that their Charter was a lie, a mean deceit, and that it would do serious damage to the London school.

Who had mounted this attack? Someone with sufficient influence to stimulate Sir James Graham — patrician autocrat — to re-examine a very recent decision by his Department. Sewell, Spooner and Simonds have been blamed. Sewell, in particular. But all three, beyond peradventure, had supported the Charter and knew its provisions. Sewell was a nonentity, and being senior of the three, the others rated even less than he did. He had been pushed around by Coleman for forty years, and part of his Professorship was to ensure that the old order continued after Coleman's death. He was certainly instructed by the Governors to sign those petitions of complaint. It was a time when noblemen could do as they wished. The opinions of three professors of a second-class calling were irrelevant. The professors must do as they were bid, or go elsewhere for patronage.

The motive? Pique. The Governors had been asked four years previously to support a charter, and had haughtily refused. Now they had been snubbed.

President Turner immediately called his Council into consultation. Sewell did not respond, but Simonds was present (a 'Mr Spooner' is in the attendance list, but in the absence of initials he cannot be identified either as Professor C. Spooner of the London school, or as the unrelated W.C. Spooner, Esq., of Southampton). The communications from the Home Office "having been read and fully considered, and this Council having taken all means in their power to ascertain the particulars referred to in such petitions, beg, agreeably to the suggestion of the Secretary of State, to transmit to him the following statement of facts . . ."

The clarity of the statement is remarkable. The Governors' objections are examined item by item. Every comment is restrained, factual and supported by documentary evidence. In particular the negotiations between the solicitors representing all parties are described in detail. Preparation of this document would have been impossible without a background of carefully preserved letters and memoranda. In all, copies of six vital documents were enclosed with the reply to Sir James Graham. In a covering letter, President Turner predicted that they would "prove the aspersions made in the two petitions to be entirely groundless." He added that, if it were considered desirable, he would be pleased to call on Sir James Graham "to substantiate the truth of the statements."

It may be recalled that President Thomas Turner and his RCVS Councillors were amateurs in the wily world of politics. They had little social standing, being of the stable rather than the drawing-room, although some read the classics and some wrote elegant prose. Only instinct could tell them what to do. Instinct served them well. It advised the unbeatable combination of simplicity and truth.

The Governors' petitions were set aside, and the RCVS continued on its way strengthened by this victory.

The next conundrum had a tartan flavour.

CHAPTER 4

Opposition from William Dick and the Edinburgh school

Surprise caused by opposition to the RCVS from the Governors of the London veterinary school, intensified to annoyance when the Highland and Agricultural Society of Scotland joined in the criticism by petitioning for a separate veterinary charter. There was collusion between London and Edinburgh in opposing the RCVS, and William Dick was involved as owner and Professor of the Edinburgh school. It seems that neither school had realised, until after the Charter had been granted, the full significance of transferring control of examinations to an independent body.

Next came examination trouble with William Dick.

The April 1844 examinations were due very soon after the Charter was granted, and the RCVS had time only to appoint for each school a temporary Board of Examiners, on which were included "those gentlemen who had already officiated for that purpose, with the addition of a certain number of veterinary surgeons in place of those disqualified as teachers from examining." Three RCVS observers attended the Edinburgh examinations: Vice-President Charles Spooner, Secretary Edmund Gabriel, and Councillor Thomas Walton Mayer.

Examinations early in the nineteenth century — so different from the hushed séances of later years — were frequently referred to as "ordeals." They were something of a Punch-and-Judy show, for not only were the victims on trial, but they were also exposed to a mixed collection of onlookers. The Edinburgh veterinary examinations of 22nd and 23rd April 1844 were held in Clyde Street Hall, the examiners being Drs Knox and Mercer of Edinburgh, Drs Macgregor and Lyon of Glasgow, and veterinary surgeons Jex of the Scots Greys, Williamson and Mather of Edinburgh, Tindall of Glasgow, Lyon of Forfar, and Thomson of Beith. Spectators included "Directors and Members of the Highland and Agricultural Society of Scotland, among whom were Sir G.M. Grant of Ballindalloch, Sir John Hope of Pinkie . . ." And so on. The examinations were verbal, and answers, feeble or bold, provided nods and smiles for a fascinated audience.

The RCVS observers, Spooner, Gabriel and Mayer were not impressed, however, and their conclusions, reported in confidence to the Council, were passed to Professor Dick. A "long correspondence ensued."

At the first Annual General Meeting of the RCVS, held in the Freemasons' Tavern on 6th May 1845, Dick asked "whether there were any reports of the proceedings on the Council to be produced." No report had, in fact, been prepared, and Mayer suggested that this should be rectified in future by publication of Council proceedings in *The Veterinarian*. Dick agreed that this would be satisfactory for the future, but he asked for an account then and there of the Council's activities during the past year; he pressed for the minutes of all meetings to be read, declaring that the profession "ought to know what the Council were doing; as, for anything they knew to the contrary, they might be doing mischief." (In parenthesis, it may be noted that as a member of the Council he could have attended all its meetings had he been so inclined.)

After a deal of discussion, Dick agreed to be satisfied by publication in *The Veterinarian* at an early date of a summary of the first year's proceedings.

This first report of the RCVS appeared in July 1845, signed by Secretary Gabriel. It provided the factual account demanded by Dick, but scarcely the material he anticipated. There was blunt criticism of the Edinburgh examinations, that were "by no means satisfactory to the Council . . . there was no examination on Chemistry — none on Materia Medica — none on Physiology — none on the Diseases of Cattle that deserved the name; there were by far too many leading questions, and the examinations were very unequal . . . the necessity of practical knowledge should be kept prominently in view in future examinations." It was recorded, further, that the pupils of the London school "passed a far better and more extended examination than their *confrères* in the North," and that the RCVS had received a memorial from "the veterinary surgeons in Glasgow" drawing attention to "the grievous state of veterinary education in the North."

Professor Dick was furious.

In a storm the elements in conflict can seem immense. When passion is spent, they can seem trifling. But storm damage so often remains. Thus with this veterinary confrontation. The ambition of the RCVS — young, eager, proud in recent recognition, determined to lead — was for *a profession*. The ambition of William Dick — self-made survivor in a hard, hard world — was for *his school*. It was naive of the RCVS to believe that hurtful criticism — however accurate — would make Dick change his ways. It was naive of Dick to dictate to a proud fledgling and expect obedience.

No sooner had battle between Dick and the RCVS been joined, than a letter was received by President Turner, headed "Whitehall, Aug. 18th, 1845," and signed, "Your obedient servant, H. Manners Sutton." The letter informed the RCVS that Home Secretary Sir James Graham had "received from various quarters, and from parties who feel a deep interest in the advancement of veterinary science, applications for the grant of a Charter of Incorporation differing, in some respects, from that which was lately granted by Her Majesty to you and certain other members of the veterinary profession."

Sir James was "disposed to attach weight to the representations." He then made the remarkable suggestion that the existing Charter should be altered in a manner that he would "be prepared on a future occasion to communicate" to the RCVS, *provided* it was first agreed "that the Charter possessed by them should undergo revision."

In reply to this astonishing proposition, the RCVS said that apart from a few individuals connected with the London and Edinburgh schools, no one had complained about the Charter and they saw no reason why it should be modified. However, "wishing to treat with the greatest respect the high source from which these intimations have emanated," they would be prepared to give "grave and mature consideration" to any amendments to the Charter that Sir James might care to suggest.

Having ruminated over this for a month, Sir James replied (through the pen of H. Manners Sutton) that nothing was closer to his heart — and to the hearts of "several important bodies" — than the "advancement of your profession." He "anxiously desired . . . that means should be found of interesting them" (i.e. the "several important bodies") "in the progress of your College, rather than that they should continue to urge hostile pretensions, which cannot but be detrimental to your prosperity, and might possibly lead to the establishment of a rival institution." He wished to reconstitute the RCVS Council by adding to it "some of the great officers of State — such as the Master of the Horse, the Master of the Buckhounds, and some of the principal medical and surgical officers of Her Majesty's forces." Sir James opined that by this blue-blood transfusion "additional dignity would be reflected on the whole professions," which would then assume "the character of a national institution," of which the "diplomas would be everywhere received with more consideration than when proceeding from a body exclusively composed of practising veterinary surgeons, as now established, however respectable."

This letter delineates with breath-taking clarity the chasms that separated early Victorian social classes. Any veterinary hope that social advancement might be part of professional recognition, was stiffly suppressed. Professional progress could only be by patronage.

The RCVS response to this suggestion is a milestone in the profession's history. Up to that moment there had been a clear professional goal. The good ship 'Charter' was on course for a land of high endeavour, where personal effort and integrity would achieve the dignity of professional recognition. Scarcely launched, the ship had met the roughest seas. Now the Home Secretary offered a safe harbour in return for a change of destination. The new landfall was to be a country where "the Master of the Horse, the Master of the Buckhounds and some of the principal medical and surgical officers of Her Majesty's forces" would lead the profession to glory.

In the words of President Turner: "In consequence of the intimation thus conveyed, that Mr Manners Sutton would be prepared to receive a deputation from your Council, your President, Messers. Percivall, Goodwin, Field, and the Secretary, were deputed to wait on that gentleman at any time that he might appoint; and, accordingly, the interview took place at the Home Office on Monday, Nov. 24, 1845: its result is contained in the following report to your Council:- 'Your President has to report, than an interview has taken place with Mr Manners Sutton, who at the commencement remarked, that he had requested it upon the understanding that the Council had agreed to certain alterations being made to the Charter. The President, however, begged to remind Mr Manners Sutton that no such acquiescence had been given. Upon which that gentleman declined entering into any particulars of the views of Sir James Graham, and the interview closed.' "

This may well be the briefest Home Office interview of all time, but it was a crucial announcement to high and low that the RCVS declined to be pushed around.

*   *   *

In the mid-1840's human and veterinary medicine achieved the new dimension of general anaesthesia. It had been known for some time that inhalation of various gases could produce giddiness, exhilaration, nausea, drowsiness: the young Humphry Davy had encountered the urge to laughter caused by nitrous oxide while the pain of surgery could be lessened by imbibed alcohol. But the concept of general anaesthesia was slow a-coming. American dentist Horace Wells was perhaps first to suggest, and to experience, surgery under general anaesthesia, when, in the autumn of 1844, one of his teeth was extracted under nitrous oxide. This kind of news travels quickly. Ether followed nitrous oxide, and chloroform followed ether. By 1847 the principles of chloroform anaesthesia were well established.

Edward Mayhew was among the first British veterinary surgeons to examine ether as a general anaesthetic. He had the unusual background of playwright and actor, being middle-aged before a passion for animal welfare led him to the London veterinary school, from which he graduated in 1845. He was a member of the "Punch" Mayhew family, Henry being the first editor of that journal and Horace a sub-editor. Edward Mayhew's considerable talents were given wholeheartedly to his new profession. He wrote well, spoke fluently and fearlessly (as a member of the RCVS council), was inventive and an acute observer. He discovered that it was possible, and relatively easy, to pass a flexible tube into the stomach of a horse via a nostril. His delight in this discovery was partly because medicines could be administered so much more easily than by mouth, but more because passing the tube was painless and barely resisted by the patient. As a comment on human silliness, it may be noted that Mayhew was so unpopular at the time for criticising the London and Edinburgh schools, that no one adopted this new technique. It was re-discovered half-a-century later. Mayhew also described how to pass a catheter in the dog, and he wrote a classic treatise on measuring the age of a horse by its teeth.

Mayhew's experiments with ether anaesthesia were typical of his offbeat approach to life. Early in 1847 *The Veterinarian* published his account of the effect of ether on a small number of dogs and cats. He recorded the clinical responses, and was satisfied that the animals were insensitive to the pain of various operations. However, he was greatly disturbed by the cries of the animals as they were losing sensibility, and when consciousness was returning. Of a cat, he wrote: "The little animal lay for six minutes and forty seconds to every appearance dead . . . I could not count the heart . . . the poor thing screamed out as it was recovering from the deadening influence." Mayhew believed that the cries were of pain. The editors of *The Veterinarian* doubted this (correctly, as it transpired), considering them to be part of the anaesthetisation process. For Mayhew, there was only one way to obtain a correct answer. He must himself be anaesthetised. With considerable difficulty, he persuaded "F. Normansell, Esq., the well-known surgeon-dentist" to administer ether and then extract a tooth. "I indicated the tooth I wished removed . . . but the gentleman . . . declared there was no disease present . . . by degrees

. . . he softened a little . . . being a medical man, he could not resist the temptation I placed before him."

Mayhew was made insensible with ether, but the good Normansell was unable to extract the tooth. As Mayhew put it: "There is, evidently, some peculiarity in the fangs, which opposes the extraction." Normansell resolutely refused to give more ether, but agreed to try to pull the tooth which had "by the force employed, been rendered sensitive." Three times he tried. This, Mayhew reported, "seemed to exhaust my endurance, and Mr Normansell kindly . . . consented to try the aether once more, on the following day." Mayhew allowed himself the luxury of a homeward journey by cab. The following day he "waited on Mr Normansell at one o'clock. Mr Rivers was present, and carefully observed me to ascertain that there was no danger in the experiment." There was no danger to Mayhew, but under the anaesthetic he wrecked the operating-room, threatened the operators, and still had his fang when he came to his senses. That evening he had "no appetite for dinner . . . and . . . was low and dull."

However, Mayhew satisfied himself that animal cries under anaesthesia were not of pain, and that "the power of aethereal vapour is a blessing to mankind."

*   *   *

The outstanding importance of the Royal Agricultural Society's financial support in 1842 for a Chair in Cattle Pathology at the London veterinary school, was amply confirmed in the years that followed. James Beart Simonds, the first Professor and veterinary adviser to the Society, received an ever-increasing number of requests for help from veterinary colleagues, land-owners, and farmers. He responded generously. He was a studious, courteous, rather serious man, restrained in speech and manner, with a flair for administration. His considerable knowledge of the diseases of farm animals was acquired from a farming background, and a practice on the outskirts of London.

It was to Simonds that Mr Statham of Datchet, near Windsor, turned for help when, in September 1847, he discovered among his sheep "a peculiar eruptive disease, accompanied with much constitutional suffering, and ending, in many cases, in . . . death."

On visiting the farm, Simonds discovered that the disease had originated among Merino sheep recently imported from Saxony and bought at Smithfield market. The first case was attributed to wasp stings, but it was soon apparent that a factor more deadly than the wasp was at work. Several deaths occurred in the next few days, and within two weeks the disease had spread to the Downland flock with which the imported animals had been mixed. The clinical signs were unfamiliar to Simonds, but he suspected that they might be of sheep-pox that he knew to be endemic on the continent of Europe. He arranged for two affected animals to be sent to the London school. One died within a few hours, and was examined *post mortem*. A medical opinion on the other was obtained from "Mr Erasmus Wilson, the. . . well-known dermatologist," who agreed with Simonds that the skin eruptions were closely similar to those of human smallpox.

Simonds now began enquiries that led eventually to the first active involvement of Government in the control of animal disease in Britain. He discovered that large numbers of sheep from the Continent "were week by week consigned to dealers in Smithfield Market . . . chiefly from Hamburg and Tonningen, and were disposed of to farmers and dealers as 'stock sheep' . . . the smallpox was spread far and wide, very many in whose systems the disease existed in its incubative stage being sent into Norfolk, where serious losses took place. Carcases were also found among low-class butchers in London who cared little as to whether the animals were free from disease or not."

Having realised, in a remarkably short time, the menace of this disease, Simonds set about attacking it. He began with the always illuminating but frequently overlooked chore of reading the literature. He found a good description by Thomas Fuller M.D. of sheep-pox in Sussex in the first decade of the eighteenth century, and noted the important conclusion that although "exceedingly contagious and mortal" among sheep, it "never infected mankind." Simonds heeded this observation and opposed those agriculturalists and medical men whose insistence that sheep-pox could be controlled by human smallpox vaccination wasted time and money and delayed eradication of the disease.

When completely satisfied that sheep-pox was a national problem that should be tackled nationally, Simonds "addressed a letter to the Board of Trade, calling attention to the fact that a disease of sheep of highly contagious and fatal nature . . . had been imported from the Continent . . . and that the animals had been sold to many farmers . . . as well as to dealers, by which the malady was widely diffused."

This letter stimulated the Government to make an Order that had "a moral influence in limiting importation." This timid beginning (understandable in a country dedicated to individual freedom) was followed by other Orders, and finally on 4th September 1848 by an Act of Parliament "to prevent the Introduction of contagious or infectious

Disorders among Sheep, Cattle, Horses and other animals." It was now official that some animals can carry some diseases around the world.

* * *

Having made the decision to oppose any attempt to modify its Charter, the RCVS adopted a firm but conciliatory attitude towards the London and Edinburgh schools. Council developed a straightforward style in discussion and correspondence that reflected calm determination to lead the profession. It was concluded that if decisions were as fair as reasonable men could devise, if government was open and dignity maintained, then, sooner or later, opponents would tire and progress would be made. To scotch any suspicion of secrecy, visitors were invited to attend Council meetings. Mr Shepperson, for example, sat in on the meeting of 19th August 1846, and Messrs Varnell, Draper, Heraud and Hooper were at the meeting of 9th February 1848. Gradually, however, this open invitation seems to have been forgotten.

The debt owed by later generations of veterinary surgeons to these early leaders is incalculable; it would have been so much easier to have gone Sir James Graham's way. President Thomas Turner and his brother James; Secretary Gabriel and Treasurer King; Councillors Braby, Arthur Cherry, Ernes, Field, Goodwin, Henderson, the Mayers father and son, Mayhew, Percivall, Robinson, W.C. Spooner and Wilkinson. Frederick Cherry, Arthur's father, is omitted from this list because he was a cross that that early Council had to bear. Although he had vigorously championed the veterinary cause back in the Coleman days, and was a regular attender at Council meetings after the Charter was obtained, he opposed virtually every motion, argued with everybody, including his son, and had good words for no one except William Dick. Time and again minutes of Council meetings record that such-and-such a decision was reached "with one exception." F.C. Cherry was the odd man out. He even refused to co-operate with his son in preparing the first register of veterinary surgeons, although as Principal Veterinary Surgeon of the Army he alone had access to the Army lists. Frederick Cherry is to be recollected, rather than remembered.

William Dick's hot reaction to RCVS criticism of the examinations at his school in 1844, shortly after the Charter had been granted, showed no sign of cooling as months went by. He missed no opportunity to criticise the Council, and did not attend its meetings. He resigned from the editorial board of *The Veterinarian*, and withdrew support from professional matters outside his school. At the second Annual General Meeting of the RCVS in 1846, he argued with the President and declared that: "He . . . had tried to act with the College; but he had been thwarted by them in every purpose he had endeavoured to work out, and he had therefore kept aloof from them for some time past."

By this time John Barlow had been appointed to teach anatomy and physiology at the Edinburgh school. Barlow, aged twenty-nine, had received his diploma from the school in 1844, and was an ardent supporter of Professor Dick. He happily undertook the role of general's aide-de-camp. However, his behaviour in support of his chief at the 1846 examinations could not be overlooked by the RCVS, however conciliatory they might wish to be. A report of the Edinburgh examinations of that year, signed by Mayhew, Gabriel and Arthur Cherry, was published in *The Veterinarian*. It noted:-

> "That the act of Professor Dick and Mr Barlow voting as 'ex officio' members of the Board of Examiners, is opposed to the express declaration of the Charter.
>
> That by interfering with the appointment of the Chairman to preside over the Board of Examiners, Professor Dick did interfere indirectly with the examinations of the pupils, and violated the intent of the Charter.
>
> That Mr Barlow, not being a Professor or an appointed Lecturer, his assumption of the right to vote as an 'ex officio' member of the Board of Examiners was a violation of the Bye-law, sect.5, 3."

Having read this in *The Veterinarian*, Barlow wrote to the RCVS, ending his letter: "I request to know on what authority it is asserted that I am not an *appointed lecturer*, and shall expect an immediate answer."

The reply to this letter, dated 30th July 1846, from Secretary Gabriel, said: "Sir, Your letter of the 11th was last night laid before the Council, and their decision is that, from its discourteous tone, it be not replied to."

Tension between William Dick and the RCVS increased. The break came in 1848. Minutes of the RCVS Council meeting of 29th March of that year record: "An official letter was read from Mr Barlow, announcing that Professor Dick had appointed a Board of Examiners for the purpose of examining his pupils."

Dick had at last carried out the threat he had made soon after the Charter was granted. He had seceded from the Royal College of Veterinary Surgeons, allowing Barlow to tell them so. His life was his school. A professional body was not his business.

CHAPTER 5

A first register of veterinary surgeons

The crisis of 1848, created by the withdrawal of Dick's school from the RCVS, was deepened by an almost simultaneous petition to Secretary of State Sir George Grey, from the Governors of the London school acting with the Highland and Agricultural Society of Scotland, for a new charter to replace that held by the RCVS. Dick's decision to break with the RCVS was influenced by support from the Highland and Agricultural Society, and by his belief that the new charter would be granted. The Royal Agricultural Society of England refused "with evident coldness" to support this application for another charter. When seeking the Society's co-operation on behalf of the Governors of the London school, Professor Sewell was asked "what it meant, as there had been one already granted by her Majesty to embody the veterinary profession." This influential support was gratefully received by a beleaguered RCVS.

In due course, however, the application for a new charter was presented to the Secretary of State. It was an arrogant document, in essence proposing that a veterinary profession should be controlled by the Professors in London and Edinburgh, acting through a Veterinary Board. The suggested constitution of the Board was reminiscent of Sir James Graham's proposal of 1845 for a reconstituted RCVS Council. True, it did not include the Master of the Buckhounds, but it did embrace "one of Her Majesty's principal Secretaries of State, or some person to be by him appointed; the president or one of the vice-presidents and three governors of the Royal Veterinary College of London; and the president, and three members of the Highland and Agricultural Society of Scotland; the principal veterinary surgeon to the army; the veterinary examiner of the Honourable East India Company; the senior professor of each of the said colleges of London and Edinburgh; and the president and vice-presidents of the to be formed new college."

The presumption of so partisan a petition was characteristic of an era when the coughs and sneezes of dukes and earls had to be treated with respect. All respect was given. It took time, of course, and earnest consultation, but eventually the petition was refused, and the RCVS breathed again.

London and Edinburgh reacted differently.

As spokesman for the London school, Professor Charles Spooner was thoroughly unpleasant at the Annual General Meeting of the RCVS in 1849, saying that "the Council had arrogated to themselves powers that they did not possess," and that their Report was "replete with inaccuracies." He said much besides, summarised by Mr Pritchard at the end of the meeting as "rubbish that ought not to have been listened to." Percivall's editorial comment in *The Veterinarian* was: "We never . . . saw the professional atmosphere convulsed by more hostile and rancorous feelings . . . the Council denounced as serving nothing but their own ends." Within a year, however, there was talk of reconciliation, and twelve months later, on the occasion of the Introductory Lecture at the London school in October 1851, "groups were seen in friendly conversation, interchanging those kindly sentiments which tend firmly to unite together the members of a common profession." Amity between the RCVS and the London school was fully forged in 1852 by the election of Professor Sewell as President RCVS. The Professor "thanked the Council for the honour conferred upon him" and "hoped that much benefit would accrue from the present amalgamation of the chartered body and the Royal Veterinary College and that no future difficulties or collision between them would ever arise."

In Edinburgh, matters followed a more convoluted course.

Having seceded from the RCVS, Professor Dick set up a Board to examine his students for a diploma of veterinary competence granted in the name of the Highland and Agricultural Society. He had no difficulty in finding medical and veterinary men to serve on this Board, for north of the Tweed sympathy was with the good Professor Dick in his battle with the English. The RCVS maintained its Board of Examiners for Scotland, and a small minority of Edinburgh students took the RCVS examination in addition to that for the Highland certificate (as it came to be called). Dick's action in ignoring the RCVS was not illegal, for there was no Act of Parliament to give bite to the Charter. In its effect, however, it was worse than illegal, for it ensured that no Act would be passed so long as he chose to dissent. Parliament would not contemplate an Act opposed by half the interested parties. The RCVS recognised the grievous consequence of losing the goodwill of Professor Dick. The only remedy was reconciliation.

A first move was made in 1850, when RCVS Secretary Gabriel visited

Edinburgh to confer with the RCVS examiners. He made contact with Professor Dick, "had several interviews . . . and received . . . an official invitation to his examination dinner." Dick "expressed the best feelings towards the Royal College of Veterinary Surgeons, and trusted that any rivalry between it and himself would be only to advance the profession; but stated that, having prevailed on the Highland and Agricultural Society to grant him a separate Board of Examiners, he could not at present secede from it." Gabriel hoped that Dick would "by and by see the desirability of doing so," and suggested that as a gesture of goodwill, the RCVS should seek Dick's advice in selecting new members for the RCVS Examining Board in Scotland.

In 1851 Gabriel nominated Dick for the RCVS Council. Unfortunately for North-South relations, he polled least votes out of twelve candidates. In 1852 there was a further twist to estrangement when Dick and Barlow wrote stuffy letters to *The Veterinarian* complaining of the inclusion of their names in the recently published RCVS Register as ex-officio members of the RCVS Board of Examiners. Dick wrote: "I do not intend to act on the Board," and Barlow echoed: "I *have not*, and shall for the future *decline to have*, any connection whatever with the Board in question."

And so on through 1853. By the end of 1854 the break was complete. Dick's horizon was the perimeter of his school, and at sixty-one authority had mutated to autocracy.

In a letter dated 31st October 1855, Secretary Gabriel — swallowing almost all RCVS pride — enquired whether Professor Dick would reconsider his secession if an "arrangement" could be made to abandon the Highland Society's certificate, and if the RCVS examination fee were reduced from ten guineas to seven. It is clear from minutes of Council meetings leading up to this letter (published in *The Veterinarian* and known to Dick), that an "arrangement" would have included retrospective recognition of the Highland Society's certificate.

Dick did not reply.

Was this the end? Could it be that there would be no Veterinary Surgeons Act, no legalised profession . . . ever?

* * *

The vital role of *The Veterinarian* in the early days of the British veterinary profession has been emphasised, and re-emphasised; it cannot be over-emphasised. Every incident in the profession's infancy was recorded and every step in childhood was noted and discussed: political aspiration and reality, clinical observation, embryonic science, the domestic scene, the doings of animals, the deeds of men. William Youatt, the gentle editor, died in 1847, mourned by all. A great, good man who gave honesty and erudition to the profession. William Percivall, founder of the journal and sole editor after Youatt's death, died in 1854. Scholar, observer, clinician, fair and fearless writer, who, to the last, obeyed his father's admonition to lead the profession by his pen. Who could follow such as these?

Not for the first time, and certainly not for the last, the veterinary profession plucked from thinnest air a man — or men — able to triumph in disaster. Had the death of Percivall been the demise, too, of *The Veterinarian*, the consequences would have been incalculable. Like obliterating newspapers. By something greater than good fortune, W.J.T. Morton and J.B. Simonds, both junior professors at the London school, took over the journal and, with no break in continuity, maintained it on its way. So skilfully did they preserve contents and format, that it is impossible to detect where the old hand was withdrawn and the new took over. Gradual changes in emphasis reflected the special interests of the new editors; Morton in chemistry, and Simonds in diseases of farm animals. Readers came to recognise whimsy in the kindly Morton's penchant for verse and the mystery of death.

*   *   *

At the RCVS Council meeting in July 1849, a satisfied Treasurer reported that money borrowed to pay Charter expenses had now been repaid (with interest), and that there was a credit balance of some £80. This stimulated Secretary Gabriel to suggest that a search should be made for "suitable apartments or a place of meeting for the College." All were agreed that a Royal College deserved a more respectable locale than the Freemasons' Tavern. T.W. Mayer donated his share of the Charter loan (some £37) "as a nucleus for the formation of a fund for the purchase of, or for building, a suitable place for the meetings of the College."

What with one thing and another, however, positive action was not taken until January 1853. A committee was then formed to acquire "rooms . . . where a museum and library could be established" with "a resident officer . . . on the spot." Several people had promised to donate "large numbers of books" to establish a library. The matter was now urgent because the Board of Examiners had become restive about "the 'improper' place (Freemasons' Tavern) at which they were compelled to conduct their examinations." After special meetings in February and

March 1853, it was resolved "that the lease of a house should be taken." In May, No. 42 Bloomsbury Square would have been acquired but for a legal technicality, but shortly afterwards No. 10 Red Lion Square was rented at £60 a-year. By January 1854 the premises were ready for occupation, the arrangement being that Secretary Gabriel would be in residence, paying £30 rent out of his £100 per annum honorarium and contributing £10 annually towards the wages of a messenger. The premises were named "The Institute of the Royal College of Veterinary Surgeons." There were many objections to "Institute", in particular, a pungent editorial in *The Veterinarian* by Percivall shortly before he died. In the event, the appellation was quietly, if gradually, forgotten.

There was still an "Institute" of the RCVS in December 1854, however, from which invitations to a *conversazione* were issued by President William Field. This first top-level party by the RCVS was a brilliant occasion. On the walls "were hung many valuable paintings by Sir E. Landseer, J. Ward R.A., and others." The tables in the council-room, board-room, library and museum were "covered with microscopes, stereoscopes and photographic drawings." There were exhibits of chemicals, and calculi, and "remarkable specimens showing the results of disease," and "rare plants from the Royal Botanic Gardens." The guests included "Professor Faraday, Sir Edwin Landseer, Sir Robert Peel, Sir Benjamin Brodie . . . Reverends . . . Professors . . . Physicians . . . Surgeons and Friends . . . Members of the Veterinary Profession." On the morning after, the organisers glowed with work well done.

*   *   *

It might have been possible to include in the Parliamentary Act required to enforce the 1844 Charter, a clause providing exemption from jury service. However, lack of co-operation from the Edinburgh school put such an Act out of the question, and an opportunity in 1851 was therefore seized to present to Parliament "a bill to exempt veterinary surgeons from serving on juries or inquests, or as churchwardens, overseers of the poor, or other parish or county officers." There was medical precedent for such exemptions, and prospects for veterinary success were good. The bill passed easily through the Lords, but was summarily rejected by the Commons. *The Veterinarian* reflected the profession's disappointment, and added: "We suspect some sinister influence has been privately at work." A second attempt to promote the bill was abandoned two years later on legal advice that "the present Government are decidedly opposed to granting any bills of examptions . . . it would be so much waste paper."

Various lists of veterinary surgeons had been compiled in the early 1800's, of lesser rather than greater accuracy. With the granting of the Charter in 1844, it became essential to have an accurate register, and an RCVS Registration Committee was formed in January 1847, with W. Arthur Cherry as Secretary. In April 1848 this Committee recommended that "for the better distinction of Members of the body corporate, the letters M.R.C.V.S. be adopted instead of V.S."

Cherry sent letters to each of the seven hundred and fifty veterinary surgeons whose address was known, asking when and from which school they had graduated, and seeking details of other people — veterinary surgeons or otherwise — treating animals in their area. The four hundred and twenty-five replies revealed that "under the various denominations of horse-doctors, horse-surgeons, farriers, cowleeches, cattle-doctors, castrators, spayers and gelders, charmers, spell-workers, butty-colliers, water-doctors, and various other local appellations, those who gain a livelihood by the practice of the art" far exceeded men who had been to veterinary school. The final estimate for the whole country was fifteen hundred graduate veterinary surgeons and six thousand others.

Cherry was designated Registrar in October 1848, and pressed on with the great task of creating a first official Register, in spite of "insults. . . . and the trouble given by nonsensical inquiries." His final report to the RCVS Council in January 1852 contained one thousand seven hundred and thirty-three names. He regretted that Edinburgh graduates of 1841 to 1844 were missing, "the returns for these years not having been placed at the disposal of the Committee when applied for." Cherry ceased to be Registrar when this work was completed, and thereafter the responsibility for maintaining the Register passed to the Secretary.

*   *   *

In April 1854 Thomas Walton Mayer resigned his seat on the RCVS Council "in consequence of increasing professional duties." His father, Thomas Mayer, a signatory to the Charter, had died in 1848. Thus ended eighteen years of unceasing endeavour by the Mayers, father and son. The veterinary profession is deeply in their debt. Mayer junior now gave up the family practice in Newcastle-under-Lyme, and joined the Army to serve in the Crimean campaign. He was one of the first British veterinary surgeons to have personal contact with cattle plague (rinderpest). In the late summer of 1855 he heard that "a dreadful murrain was destroying immense numbers of cattle in Asiatic Turkey . . . and in a few weeks the disease made its appearance in our camp . . . I at once perceived that I had to deal with a disease of no ordinary character." Mayer's experiences with cattle plague were published in *The Veterinarian* in the spring of 1857, accompanied by an editorial in which Morton and Simonds said: "We wish in an especial manner to direct the attention of our readers to the circumstance that a most destructive cattle epizootic, new to the present generation of Englishmen, will probably ere long be introduced into this country from the Continent . . . the circumstance does not take us by surprise, for, from the time it was ascertained that the malady was existing in the Crimea, Turkey, and adjacent countries during the late war, we felt assured it would extend to those Kingdoms and States where it had been unknown, except by name, for years." The editors gave the history of the last outbreak of the disease in Britain (ending in 1757), and emphasised that it must be differentiated from pleuro-pneumonia, a chronic disease of cattle imported into Britain about 1840. Cattle plague was not just an acute form of pleuro-pneumonia, as suggested by "many agriculturalists, and not a few medical men of eminence." The editorial ended by urging that veterinary surgeons be consulted about the control of this and other animal diseases.

This hint (undoubtedly from Simonds's pen, for Morton was a chemist) may have been taken, for Simonds was invited to visit the European Continent to assess the threat of cattle plague to the United Kingdom, his expenses to be shared by the Royal Agricultural Society of England, the Highland and Agricultural Society of Scotland, and the Royal Agricultural Improvement Society of Ireland. William Ernes, a Belgian veterinary surgeon long settled in Britain, master of several European languages, was to be his travelling companion and interpreter. The journey began on 9th April 1857. Professor Dick, consulted by the Highland and Agricultural Society, had opposed the proposal to send Simonds across the Channel, because: "I considered such a mission to be unnecessary, as we would get every information regarding the disease from the veterinary surgeons on the Continent . . . I apprehended Professor Simonds's journey would prove to be a kind of wild-goose chase."

Wild-goose chase or no, Simonds's investigation was an important episode in British veterinary history. The journeying was extensive, examination of the problem was thorough, and the immediate report was a first-class account of all aspects of the disease. Those responsible for commissioning Simonds were impressed. Veterinary epidemiology and preventive medicine in Britain were in the making.

Carrying letters of introduction from the Foreign Office to "British Consular Agents in Northern and Central Europe," Simonds and Ernes visited Belgium, Holland, Westphalia and Hanover, Denmark, Schleswig, Holstein, Lübeck, Mecklenburg-Schwerin, Mecklenburg-Strelitz, Saxony, Prussia, Silesia, Galicia, Austria, Bavaria, and Wurtemburg. They were instructed on the history and control of diseases of cattle in each country; they visited farms and dairies; they talked with all manner of people, especially veterinarians, farmers and cattle dealers. Four facts were soon established. First, that the authorities in every country knew more about cattle plague than their opposite numbers in Britain. Secondly, that they were terrified of the disease. Thirdly, that they would take the most stringent precautions to control it, including standstill areas and slaughter of affected and in-contact animals. Fourthly, that at that time there was no cattle plague in Northern or Western Europe.

Simonds was determined to see the disease, however, so they travelled eastwards towards the Polish frontier. A month after leaving London they made contact with an outbreak in Galicia and were permitted, at the quarantine stations, to follow the course of the disease, hour by hour, in eight animals, and to carry out post mortem examinations.

Simonds's long report (ten instalments in *The Veterinarian*) ended with sixteen crisp, summarising paragraphs, concentrating especially on field control of the disease. The final conclusion was that because of the remoteness of infected areas and the Draconian measures taken to control the disease on the continent, "no fear need be entertained that this destructive pest will reach our shores." That this conclusion referred only to that particular time and the circumstances then pertaining, is made clear in a Morton editorial in *The Veterinarian* praising the report: ". . . since the time may come — although there is no fear at present — when this formidable malady will reach our shores through the introduction of foreign cattle."

*   *   *

There appeared in *The Veterinarian* for April 1855: " 'Historical and Critical Remarks on Nasal Polypus.' By J. Gamgee, M.R.C.V.S., London." It began: "The learned Adams, in his Commentaries on 'The Seven Books of Paulus Aegineta,' says, that 'Hippocrates describes five species of polypus . . . Galen gives various 'prescriptions from Archigenes, Asclepiades, Lampon, and others, for removing polypus . . .' Antonio Musa recommends . . . Celsus, Oribasius, Scribonius, Octavius Horatianus, Aëtius, Alexander, Marcellus, and amongst the Arabians, Serapion, Albucasis, Avicenna . . ."

Names dropped like daisies across a meadow, the reader entranced, irritated, or stunned by a torrent of words. The author was veterinary surgeon John Gamgee, aged twenty-five, graduate from the London school in 1852; son of Joseph Gamgee, veterinary surgeon; born and reared in Italy; artist, linguist; second of three brilliant brothers. He has a special place in British veterinary history for the manner in which he stimulated all around him, during a professional life of only sixteen years. Folk were either fascinated or infuriated; no one was neutral.

Gamgee, a European, familiar with continental veterinary schools, contributed to *The Veterinarian* abstracted translations entitled "Contemporary Progress of Veterinary Science and Art." When John Barlow died in 1856, Dick appointed Gamgee to succeed him as Professor of Anatomy and Physiology. They parted after twelve explosive months. Dick maintained: "I engaged him for one year only." In fact, the most liberal offering to Dick and his school by this brash young man was continuous criticism. There can be sympathy with Dick in bending before a whirlwind.

Faithful to his make-up, when Gamgee left Dick's school he founded a New Veterinary College — not in Bradford, Liverpool or Inverness, but right there, under Dick's nose, in Drummond Street, Edinburgh.

Dick had no fear of rivalry from this upstart lecturer. At least, not until he realised that Gamgee had applied for affiliation by Sign Manual to the RCVS.

CHAPTER 6

John Gamgee's school in Edinburgh

Among persons covered by the Charter of 1844, were "such . . . of our loving subjects as . . . may hereafter become students of the Royal Veterinary College of London, or of the Veterinary College of Edinburgh, or of such other Veterinary College . . . as . . . shall be established for the purposes of education in veterinary surgery . . . in our United Kingdom, and which we, or our Royal successors, shall under our or their sign manual authorise."

John Gamgee's application, dated 7th April 1858, for affiliation of his New Edinburgh school with the RCVS by Royal Sign Manual, was the first of its kind. The result would be a precedent, and must be carefully considered. A good impression created by the profusion of signatures of Scottish Nobility, Professors and Gentlemen appended to the application — reflecting Gamgee's personal magnetism, for he had been but a short time in Scotland — was offset by the acute antagonism of William Dick, backed by the Highland and Agricultural Society.

In May, in reply to a request for an opinion on Gamgee's application, the RCVS stated that "the Charter did not confer on the council the power to interfere with the schools." They dared not say openly how much they wished the application to succeed, lest Dick's wrath be transferred to them from Gamgee.

In a letter dated 7th July, addressed to the Under Secretary of State for the Home Department, John Hall Maxwell, on behalf of the Highland and Agricultural Society, wrote: "The new Veterinary College or School of Edinburgh is simply a private class unconnected with any public body in Edinburgh or Scotland, and it is very questionable how far it is provided with the staff, buildings, and general plant or appendages which are essential to a college . . . the only legitimate grounds on which a new college could be recognised would be the inefficiency of the existing institution. Professor Dick, its founder and head . . . by his energy, perseverance and liberality . . . has, single-handed, and at a personal outlay of above ten thousand pounds . . . sent forth nearly 600 veterinarians . . . to practise their art."

The application was refused shortly after the date of this letter, essentially on the basis of its contents.

This verdict was unacceptable to Gamgee's sponsors, in particular to James Syme, Professor of Clinical Surgery at the Edinburgh medical school. He circularized members of the Highland and Agricultural Society, describing Gamgee as "a gentleman of remarkable talent, extensive acquirements, and personal qualities of no ordinary kind," and emphasising what he considered to be the iniquity of the Home Department decision. He said of the alleged perfection of Dick's school: "I have been accustomed to hear opinions of an entirely different kind," and he challenged the conclusion that "it was not for the interest of veterinary instruction in Scotland that Mr Gamgee should be allowed to compete in teaching with Mr Dick."

Replying to this circular, Dick minced none of two thousand words. He attacked Syme ("my assailant"), Gamgee, and the New College with its financial fulcrum of a joint-stock company.

This bickering between individuals of local reputation but national nonentity, set a problem for the Home Department who had reached a decision and were reluctant to recant. The Lord Advocate of Scotland turned to the RCVS for guidance, but after a meeting with Secretary Gabriel on 28th February 1859, it could only be concluded that: "The responsibility of granting the Sign Manual rested on Her Majesty's Government, and the responsibility of the Examinations on the Board of Examiners."

The RCVS refused to be involved. They already had more than enough opposition from Professor Dick.

The outcome?

A revised decision by the Home Department.

The Royal Sign Manual for affiliation of John Gamgee's New Edinburgh veterinary school with the RCVS was granted on 31st March 1859.

The significance of this ruling was great. It dissipated for ever the myth that only one school in England and one in Scotland could provide veterinary education. It recognised beyond peradventure that the RCVS was the legal ruling body of a veterinary profession to which all schools must be affiliated. It was *de facto* predication that Professor Dick's Highland certificate of veterinary competence did not conform with the provisions of the 1844 Charter. If that Charter were to acquire Parliamentary backing, Dick's certificate would be without value as a professional qualification.

All this was understood by John Gamgee. It was his most important contribution to the British veterinary profession.

*   *   *

Thomas Turner, named in the 1844 Charter as first President of the RCVS, died in 1859 aged sixty. It can sincerely be echoed from his obituary in *The Veterinarian* that "none more anxiously laboured for the benefit of the profession." Turner's gentlemanly bearing and integrity were invaluable in the profession's earliest days. Due to poor health, he relinquished the Presidency in 1851. A subscription was opened to have his portrait painted. This, the first of many cherished pictures of past Presidents, executed by W. Pickersgill, Esq., R.A. and of kitcat size, was presented to the Council in October 1855. It was said: "No one can look at it without being struck with its resemblance to the original, even though there be a little of the artist's allowed flattery — juvenility — in it." Most Presidents after Thomas Turner have held office for one year only, but there have been exceptions related to exceptional circumstances.

Another trusted servant, Secretary Edmund Gabriel, was lost to the RCVS in 1861. Persistent ill-health forced him to resign, to be replaced, briefly, by Edward Braby, and then by William Henry Coates, both veterinary surgeons, working, as Gabriel had done, for an honorarium. Gabriel died in 1864. As with Thomas Turner, his honesty, good manners, and allround ability were of inestimable value in the early negotiations with Authority, when the precious Charter might so easily have slipped away. As one of the RCVS observers (with Thomas Walton Mayer and Charles Spooner) at the fateful first examination in Edinburgh in 1844, Gabriel accepted his share of the responsibility for criticising Professor Dick. In honesty he could not have done otherwise, but no one strove harder to heal the breach that followed. His pleasure was great at the affiliation between the RCVS and Gamgee's school, because he knew that it was the first move back to unity.

*   *   *

The manner in which editors Morton and Simonds of *The Veterinarian* continued the Percivall/Youatt tradition of keeping readers in touch with scientific progress, is no more strikingly demonstrated than in their editorials on Pasteur's classic writings on spontaneous generation, fermentation and putrefaction in the early 1860's. They understood the significance of Pasteur's experiments when applied to infectious diseases, and were anxious to spread the news of a satisfactory explanation for the apparently inexplicable. Disease did not arise spontaneously in dirt or dung, but was caused by a living *something* to be detected only by a microscope. The acceptance by Morton and Simonds of Pasteur's early conclusions, was by no means typical of the time. Indeed, agnostics and disbelievers were still at large two decades later. To emphasise the application of this new knowledge in the veterinary field, Simonds wrote of the outbreak of sheep-pox in Berkshire in 1862: "It is satisfactory to know that the advocates of the spontaneous origin of the disease have little or no ground for their theory in its spread." Extension of the outbreak was due to "the established traffic in sheep, which at this period of the year is more than ordinary in the western counties." In short, affected sheep passed the disease to healthy sheep.

Acute editorial interest in the concept of minute living particles being involved in biological processes, can be sensed in *The Veterinarian* for 1864: "The Origin of Infusoria." Experimental evidence — much by Pasteur — was examined, and the point was made that "scarcely anything is known concerning these minute organisms," referred to as "Bacteriums"; thought by some to be animals, by others to be vegetables, and by Mr H.J. Clark, of Cambridge, U.S. to be "nothing more than portions of decomposed muscular fibre or tissue." The editorial conclusion was that: "It is not honest to take no account of facts that contradict our own notions, to cite Pasteur, and omit Pouchet or Wyman. As the matter really stands, there are discrepancies which have to be explained."

A conclusion beyond dispute.

In 1864, too, *The Veterinarian* published a translation by W. Ernes, MRCVS (who had accompanied Simonds seven years previously on his cattle plague investigation across Europe), of "Researches on the Infusoria of the Blood in the Malady known as Apoplexy of the Spleen," by Casimir Davaine, a French doctor of medicine. Apoplexy of the spleen — anthrax — is a rapidly lethal disease in animals, and is sometimes fatal in man. In this paper, Davaine recalled that in 1850 he and the French physician Pierre Rayer had seen in the blood of two sheep that had died of anthrax microscopic "filiform bodies double the length of blood globules." Davaine had intended to search for these bodies in other animals that had died of anthrax, but did not actually do so until eleven years later when, stimulated by Pasteur's suggestion that microorganisms were involved in fermentation, he found in the blood of another sheep dead of anthrax "an immense number of Bacteria . . . exactly like those I had observed in 1850." He guessed, but could not prove, that the filiform bodies were the cause of the disease. He said: "Doctors in medicine and naturalists have theoretically admitted that contagious maladies, epidemic fevers, the pest, &c., are determined by invisible animalcula or ferments; but I am not aware that any positive observation has ever confirmed their views."

Although Davaine could not prove that anthrax was caused by bacteria, he guessed that the delay between infection of an animal and the appearance of clinical disease (the so-called incubation period, already well recognised for several diseases), could be explained by the time taken for an invading "animalcule" to multiply to a noxious level.

For Morton and Simonds — and many, many others — excitement in Davaine's discoveries was intense.

Faithful to its readers, however, *The Veterinarian* kept scientific matters in perspective by reporting not only Casimir Davaine, but also a less esoteric aspect of the lore of the land. In 1863 "a respectable-looking woman . . . with . . . a child about six" applied to the Clerkenwell magistrate for destruction of a dog that had bitten the child. She declared that "a fortune-teller had said that the dog had better be killed, or else her child would go mad . . . when the planets crossed such a thing might occur." The magistrate said "foolish twaddle," and decided that the dog should live. The woman had to accept his ruling, but commented that she "would see what a little dose of poison upon some nice meat would do for the brute of a dog that had bitten her child."

*   *   *

By chance, speakers at the RCVS Annual Dinner in the Freemasons' Tavern on 4th May 1863 combined to present in microcosm a contemporary picture of the veterinary profession. After loyal toasts to the Queen and the Prince and Princess of Wales, President J.B. Simonds proposed "The Duke of Cambridge and the Army." He said: "You are all mindful . . . that the army is a means by which very many of the members of our profession find employment, and are introduced into the very best society." The Principal Veterinary Surgeon to the Army, J. Wilkinson, replying, confirmed that "great improvements . . . in our army establishment . . . have enabled me to offer better terms to . . . candidates if we could only improve . . . primary education . . . we should hold a high position in society." He added: "Many persons who now enter the medical profession, having a love for horses, would come into ours, only that they do not like the idea of going a step down instead of keeping on a level . . . they have already reached."

W. Ernes proposed "The College of Physicians and the College of Surgeons." He rejoiced in the progress made by these Colleges. He sometimes attended their public lectures. He hoped that "the time will come when the College of Veterinary Surgeons will have a place where occasionally lectures can be delivered, and that they may also investigate scientific matters." In reply, Mr Quain saw no reason "why there should not be the greatest possible sympathy between the College of Veterinary Surgeons and the College of Physicians, and the Royal College of Surgeons. Their anatomy is very nearly the same, their physiology is quite identical, their pathology also."

A toast, to "The Court of Examiners" recalled the Coleman days when all examiners were medical men, followed after the 1844 Charter by a mixture of medical men and veterinary surgeons who had worked well together. It was said of some veterinary students that "in anatomy and physiology they answer . . . as well as any men who go to the College of Physicians or the College of Surgeons."

In reply to personal well-wishing, RCVS President Simonds recalled his appointment some twenty years earlier to the London school, to teach the then new subject of diseases of farm animals. He deplored the small number of members attending the Annual Meeting (as almost every RCVS President has done almost every year since 1844). He remembered President Field's brilliant *conversazione*, and regretted that no other President — himself included — had succeeded in repeating so successful an enterprise. He was pleased to have the company that evening of medical colleagues, and he had high hopes for veterinary science in the future.

The toast to "The Schools and Teachers" was coupled with the name of Professor Gamgee, who, in an effervescent reply, hoped that "the day was not far distant when veterinary colleges would have a better opportunity of doing justice to themselves and to the students." He suggested summer sessions at the schools, and a "course of instruction . . . over three years instead of two."

Then the mature and reassuring Dr Sharpey, Professor of Physiology at University College, London, a non-veterinary member of the Court of Examiners, proposed "The Veterinary Profession." Aware of the difficulties created by unqualified practitioners and holders of Professor Dick's Highland certificate, Dr Sharpey referred to the "feeling of reproach that, of all the persons engaged in the practice of the veterinary profession, only about a third have received testimonials of fitness from the Royal College of Veterinary Surgeons." But, he observed wisely, "all professions have to go through certain stages of progress." Herbalists and barbers had begotten physicians and surgeons. Handicraftsmen became professionals. A new era had been opened for the veterinary profession "by the institution and by the labours of the Royal College of Veterinary Surgeons." Dr Sharpey considered it "a pleasure to be associated in the task of elevating the veterinary profession . . . now fairly launched . . . in a line of advancement which cannot fail to place it high in the public estimation."

W. Robinson proposed "The Royal Agricultural Society," recalling astonishing progress since "its first meeting in Oxford, where, amongst the animals exhibited, there was but a single sire, and the implements comprised two or three carts and waggons, and a few machines employed in agriculture."

Replying to "The Country Practitioners," W. Burley contrasted "the difficulty of obtaining veterinary instruction in his youthful days with the facilities at present afforded by the veterinary schools."

G.T. Brown, for thirteen years veterinary professor at the Cirencester College of Agriculture, replied to "The Vice-Presidents and Stewards." He regretted the "lamentable want of preliminary education in the students who presented themselves at the schools," and called for "mutual forbearance" on the part of the medical and veterinary professions.

The Secretary of the RCVS, W.H. Coates, was toasted, and complimented particularly on the improved Register, with its County and Military lists.

At last: "The toast of the ladies having, at the instance of Mr. C. Dickens, been duly honoured, the company separated about 11 o'clock."

The ladies did not participate, of course, in that RCVS Dinner. Nor did they, indeed, for another nine-and-seventy years.

*   *   *

The year 1865 was momentous in British veterinary history. In the early summer cattle plague entered the country (probably from Russia), killed an estimated half million cattle, and was eventually controlled by veterinary procedures which, although advised from the start, were only accepted when every other method had failed. The present Animal Health Division of the Ministry of Agriculture, Fisheries & Food dates from that time.

Clearly, the individuals who controlled this devastating disease deserve an honourable place in history.

For this reason, a digression even in this brief history is unavoidable. Major-General Sir Frederick Smith whose monumental labours on behalf of British veterinary history are enshrined in several publications, but especially in four volumes of "The Early History of Veterinary Literature," has given all credit for controlling cattle plague in Britain to John Gamgee. Of James Beart Simonds, veterinary adviser to the Royal Agricultural Society and the Privy Council at the time, Sir Frederick has written: "His public professional life was ruined by his belief in spontaneous generation." And: ". . . it was to him, and a Government bent on free trade even in disease, that the invasion of Cattle Plague in 1865 was due."

Examination of contemporary literature, official reports, and minutes of Privy Council proceedings has failed to reveal the basis for Sir Frederick's strictures on Simonds and support for Gamgee. Indeed, it has been concluded that Simonds deserves major credit for handling officialdom and eliminating cattle plague, and that John Gamgee played the minor role of publicist for control measures already advocated and fully understood by Simonds and others.

No explanation has been found for Sir Frederick's contention that Simonds believed that cattle plague could arise spontaneously. As this statement is seriously damaging to Simonds's reputation, and casts doubt on the reliability of the advice he gave to the Privy Council, the following questions and answers are quoted from the Commission of Enquiry into the origin of the disease. The date is October 1865. Simonds is answering questions put by Viscount Cranbourne. The questions are numbered 255 to 257:-

"255. You believe that the whole of southern Russia is the seat of the spontaneous generation of this disease? — I do not believe that it has a spontaneous origin anywhere. I believe that the whole of the southern part of Russia is the home of the pest, and that it always abides there. 256. Do you mean to say that it originally made its appearance there? — I cannot say that, or whether it came from Asia, or whether it is a continuance of the plague that fell upon the Egyptians; I think that we know no more of the origin of this disease than we do of the origin of small-pox or the cholera. 257. Do you believe that there is no instance of the spontaneous generation of this disease? — I believe so."

From the time of his visit to the European Continent with Ernes in

1857, Simonds took a special interest in cattle plague, reporting in *The Veterinarian* its presence in various countries. Thus, in 1860 it was "raging to a fearful extent" in Galicia, and "its extension towards the Prussian frontier from Austro-Poland is creating great anxiety." In 1862 it was introduced into southern Italy "by some Illyrian oxen, disembarked either at Louciano or Foggio." In 1863 it was "making great ravages in . . . the Austrian dominions," and there were reports that sheep were affected. In 1864 there was a "great spread of the cattle disease throughout the Roman States." Simonds was also lecturing on the disease to his students, one of whom (Thomas Walley, later Principal of the Edinburgh veterinary school) recorded that in 1861 Professor Simonds "emphatically declared his conviction that nothing could save this country from a visitation of the disease, unless the authorities realised the probability of such a contingency arising and adopted vigorous measures to prevent it."

Besides being aware of the threat to Britain from cattle plague in the early 1860s, Simonds was concerned by the unpreparedness of the country to meet the danger. His considerable experience of the working of government, however, and an interest in the mechanics of administration, made him realise the difficulty of legislating against calamity in prospect. Would Englishmen tolerate restriction of their liberty to buy and sell cattle from and to whom they wished? He doubted it. He considered the possibility of a hostile public in an editorial in the April number of *The Veterinarian* for 1860, entitled: "Necessity of Legislative Enactments to Limit the Spread of Contagious Diseases Among Cattle," and urged collection of statistics on which realistic legislation could be based. He wrote: "The governmental . . . machinery is at hand . . . to this could easily be added a veterinary section for . . . receiving returns and . . . carrying into practice . . . sanitary measures . . . necessary to preserve the health of those animals which furnish food and clothing to our people."

Simonds' advice, to his colleagues and the country, on the potential danger of cattle plague, may be described as measured and muted compared with the cataract of propaganda that poured from John Gamgee's pen. Shortly after starting his school in Edinburgh, Gamgee launched *The Edinburgh Veterinary Review* to give literary scope to a bubbling brain. A favourite subject — extended to the newspapers — was the vulnerability of Britain to infectious diseases. What Gamgee said was, in essence, no different from what Simonds was saying, but it was announced with such a flourish that the impression was created in many minds that only John Gamgee understood infectious disease and could preserve the country.

It is possible that Sir Frederick Smith was deceived by this welter of words.

Be that as it may, Simonds and Gamgee, each in his own way, warned Britain of trouble if cattle plague reached her shores.

CHAPTER 7

The cattle plague disaster of 1865

The cattle plague epidemic of 1865/66 is one of the most extensively documented episodes in British veterinary history. It could scarcely be otherwise. The disease is so infectious and so rapidly fatal and Britain was so vulnerable, that everyone was involved. From the dairymaid without a cow to milk, to the Archbishop of Canterbury seeking the ear of the Almighty: "We acknowledge our transgressions, which worthily deserve Thy chastisement . . . stay, we pray Thee, this plague . . . shield our homes from its ravages . . . Amen."

The saga of the epidemic can be comprehensively followed from the official reports. It is a long read, but complete in the detail of who did what, and what happened when. Veterinary angles can be measured from evidence given during two weeks in October 1865, to a Governmental committee of twelve Cattle Plague Commissioners. Forty-four individuals were examined, including fifteen British veterinary surgeons, and a deputation from the City of London. The examination of James Beart Simonds and William Ernes (interviewed together) occupied all the first day; John Gamgee appeared a week later, William Dick the day after Gamgee.

Simonds described to the Commissioners the first suspected case: "On the 4th of July, Mr Priestman, a veterinary surgeon living near to the Metropolitan Cattle Market, and Mr Nichols, the son of Mrs Nichols, who has a large dairy in Islington, came to the Veterinary College, bringing with them the stomach and intestines of a cow, they being under the impression that the animal had died of poison." Simonds visited the dairy, saw other sick animals, and "came . . . to the conclusion that they were dying from a . . . disease having many of the characters" of cattle plague. However, "there were some points of difference which required investigation, for example, there was not the same amount of discharge from the eyes . . . nor the same nervous twitchings . . . that we had observed in Galicia."

This variability in the early clinical picture of cattle plague has caused diagnostic difficulty on other occasions, a point emphasised in John Gamgee's evidence to the Commissioners. He said: "It is very strange that the disease presents singular symptoms in different countries."

Simonds told veterinary surgeon Priestman that he suspected cattle plague, also his colleague at the London school G.W. Varnell who had seen organs from the first case, but he did not report to the Privy Council until six days later. He informed the Commissioners: "It was on the morning of the 10th of July that I called the attention of the Privy Council to the matter; my attention having been first called to it on the afterpart of the 4th of July. I occupied five days in investigating the matter thoroughly to my own satisfaction, and on the 9th of July my mind was made up."

The minutes of a Privy Council meeting on 10th July 1865 record: "In consequence of information received at the Council office that a disease of malignant character was prevalent among cows in the London dairies, the Lord President directed Professor Simonds to at once institute an enquiry."

In parenthesis, it may be noted that use of the description "a disease of malignant character," instead of "cattle plague," has been held against Simonds, suggesting that he did not recognise the disease. This is unjust. He was a cautious man. Far better to be careful at first, and correct in the end. It was a repetition of his first diagnosis of sheep-pox many years before. A wrong diagnosis of cattle plague could have caused great harm.

Simonds was now officially in charge, and the Council awaited his advice. It was an awesome responsibility. No administrative machinery, and dying and dead cattle everywhere. It had become clear that the disease had been in the country for some time, the probable origin being a cargo of live cattle from the Baltic port of Revel, off-loaded at Hull.

Simonds reported to the Council on 13th July, urging as a first step an immediate Order in Council to control movement of cattle and to assess the extent of the epidemic. The next day: "Their Lordships directed that the Law Officers of the Crown should be instructed to prepare a draft Order, as suggested." The Order was ready ten days later, and at a meeting of the Council on 24th July: "Their Lordships . . . having received further particulars . . . from Professor Simonds, were pleased" to give their approval.

It is unnecessary to follow in detail the story over the turbulent months that followed, for it has often been told. Suffice it to say that the advice of Simonds and Gamgee to restrict movement and to slaughter affected animals was ignored. Both knew from personal experience on the European continent that treatment was useless, and that only the most rigorous "stamping-out" policy could eliminate the disease. But medical men (with a few notable exceptions), and the general public, knew nothing of infectious diseases in animals, and could not grasp the concept of slaughtering an animal to protect its fellows. They were so used to the idea of treatment, that to kill seemed the ultimate in callous ignorance. The cry was for sanataria and treatment. Newspapers were vociferous. The veterinary profession was cast into the pit.

So the disease spread to all corners of the country. Wherever it appeared cattle died in staggering numbers. In September Simonds diagnosed the disease in sheep, and they too died. Small wonder that the Archbishop's prayer had a sense of urgency about it.

John Gamgee's evidence to the Cattle Plague Commissioners was excellent, although he had to admit that he had not reached London and actually seen the disease until 29th July (by which time it was well recognised by everybody, the first Order in Council was almost a week old, and Simonds had produced the disease experimentally at the London veterinary school, by placing a healthy cow in contact with an affected animal on 13th July, and seeing the healthy animal sicken ten days later). Gamgee had been caught unawares by the actual arrival of cattle plague, after having forecast its coming, probably from Russia, as far back as 1863. His New veterinary school in Edinburgh was in financial difficulty (losing a thousand pounds annually), and he was in the process of transferring it to London, where, after a monetary transfusion, it was to re-emerge as the "Royal Albert Veterinary College." An intimate glimpse of John Gamgee is given in his public notice of this change of venue for the school:-

> "It is proposed to transfer to London the New Veterinary College of Edinburgh, presided over, under 'Royal Sign Manual,' by Professor Gamgee, whose ability and eminent services to the advancement of veterinary science have acquired a widespread reputation. Professor John Gamgee has been solicited and induced to accede to a preliminary arrangement, whereby his whole staff of professors, teachers, and students, museum, library, diagrams, apparatus &c., shall be secured for the London College."

Here, if ever, was virtue in necessity.

In contrast to the expert opinion of Simonds and Gamgee, William Dick's evidence to the Cattle Plague Commissioners makes embarrassing reading. Asked about steps taken in Edinburgh, he described a

sanatarium where diseased animals were treated. "I commence . . . by the administration of mild purgatives, followed by stimulants, and after that, tonics . . . where the disease has been a little more advanced . . . a dose of oil . . . lime water and tincture of opium."

"Do you see your way to the end of this disease, or do you see any chance of getting rid of it? — I do think that in a little time it will disappear.
What is it that you rely upon? — Upon a change in the weather."

At which point a curtain may tactfully be drawn to deaden discussion of abundant flies in Scotland that summer, and obnoxious vapours rising from burns near byres.

As treatment after treatment proved useless, as weeks stretched into months, and as the massacre continued, it began to dawn on even the most prejudiced that veterinary advice might be heeded. The influence of the Royal Agricultural Society, with Simonds their adviser, was crucial in persuading the country to adopt the continental slaughter policy. Once the principle of slaughter instead of treatment was accepted, the Cattle Diseases Prevention Act was speedily prepared and approved. It became law in February 1866, and its success may be gauged from the fact that whereas some 18,000 new cases of cattle plague were notified in one week of that month, only eight were reported in one week nine months later.

In eighteen hectic months cattle plague revolutionised the British veterinary profession. Before June 1865 disease was treated on a single-animal basis, with the horse by far the most usual patient. There was minimal Government interest in animal welfare, except in the specialised military world, and veterinary surgeons were seen as men who treated lameness or colic. Suddenly all was changed. The profession had saved the country. It had a new status, a special place in the life of the Nation.

At a very early stage in the epidemic, it became clear that letters, queries, instructions and the like must pass through a central point. The obvious clearing house was the Privy Council office, and a veterinary department was established. This was the beginning of a Government veterinary service in Britain. The whole profession was involved in the cattle plague epidemic, because inspectors were required to implement the control measures in the Orders and the Act that eliminated the disease. This was a new veterinary service to the community, a new veterinary dimension.

John Gamgee's part in the epidemic ended with the publication in 1866 of a tome entitled, "The Cattle Plague." The purpose of this volume is obscure, for it contains very little indeed that is original. It is written as if no one but Gamgee knew anything about cattle plague. Much space is given to reports of the International Veterinary Congresses at Hamburg in 1863 and Vienna in 1865, in which Gamgee played a leading role. Gamgee's prophetic writings on cattle plague are given *in extenso*, and he alleges that he had "to bear up against torrents of abuse, imputations as to motives, and gross misrepresentations." The most interesting section is an account of measurement of temperatures in cattle plague by Gamgee and his brother Arthur, among the earliest observations on veterinary clinical thermometry. A black mark for Gamgee is his accusation that Simonds did not recognise cattle plague when it reached Britain. This untruth is unworthy of an exceptional mind. It was a mind under pressure, however, and the clue to this enigmatic volume may be in the Prospectus for the Albert Veterinary College, Queen's Road, Bayswater, bound in at the back. Gamgee's financial difficulties may explain why "The Cattle Plague" reads like an overgrown advertising brochure.

The Albert Veterinary College failed two years later, and Gamgee forsook veterinary science, turning his talents to research on refrigeration and the international transport of frozen meat. He spent but sixteen years in the veterinary world, and was only thirty-seven when he sought new pastures. For some he was arrogant beyond endurance, but his golden tongue, his facile pen and his intellectual brilliance stimulated and enriched the profession.

*   *   *

Pre-dating, coincident with, and post-dating the epidemic of cattle plague, the proposition of a Veterinary Medical Bill harassed the RCVS Council from 1863 to 1867. It is a story of high hope, prolonged negotiation, and ultimate frustration. There is a dispiriting inevitability about the tale, that began with the discovery in 1862/63 in the United Kingdom of 1,018 Members of the RCVS, 1,244 unqualified persons calling themselves veterinary surgeons, and 1,189 others engaged in veterinary practice in various disguises. This was intolerable. It was agreed to prepare "a Petition to Parliament, with a view to obtain an Act for the better protection of Members of the Body Corporate."

The draft of a Bill was discussed by the RCVS Council on 14th October 1863, approved, and passed to "Mr Garrard, the legal adviser of the College, for his opinion and with a view . . . of ascertaining the cost and . . . the necessary steps to be taken." Mr Garrard advised, and the Council agreed, that the opinion of Counsel should be obtained "as to the probability of the Bill being passed through the House." The Bill had two objectives. First, to limit the title of veterinary surgeon to Members of the RCVS. Secondly, to exempt Members of the RCVS "from serving on all Juries and Inquests whatsoever."

The original intention was a Private Bill, but time was lost in "mature consideration, and in obtaining legal opinions," and eventually in 1864 President Ernes tried to arrange for a Public Bill. On legal advice it was to be prospective only, meaning that anyone calling himself a veterinary surgeon at the time of passing the Act could continue to use that title. No progress had been made by the time of the 1864 RCVS Annual General Meeting; hope had been abandoned that the Government would adopt the Bill, and President Ernes made the ominous comment that: "The Council at first eagerly adopted . . . every clause in the Bill . . . then, for some reason, I cannot tell what, the Council altered their opinion, and seemed rather afraid of proceeding with the Bill."

A year of inaction followed. President Hunt made no reference to the Bill in his Annual Report, and it is not surprising that William Ernes, President the previous year, was sharply critical of the delay.

By this time, however, even the dimmest eyes could read between the lines. If the Bill became law, those who thereafter obtained Professor Dick's Highland certificate could not call themselves veterinary surgeons.

On a date that has not been determined, but probably towards the end of 1865, William Dick received a Memorial signed by seventy-one men who had attended his school and had received his Highland certificate. Army officers were included, and some of the best-known practitioners in the Kingdom. This remarkable document reveals the extent to which Professor Dick's refusal to cooperate with the RCVS for twenty-two years, in spite of every size of olive branch, had brought the profession to its knees. These men, his own students, proud of their Alma Mater and its "Venerable Head," as they described him, begged "that it may please you to enter into negotiations at once with the Council of the Royal College of Veterinary Surgeons, for the re-arranging by them of the Examining Board of the Edinburgh Veterinary College, and at the same time make such honorable arrangements as will enable those of us who hold the Diploma of the Edinburgh College only to obtain the Chartered one . . . your Memorialists are anxious you should take this step from a sincere desire for the well-being, prosperity, and permanence of the Institution with which your name has been associated, with so much credit and justly earned fame, from its birth to the present time."

No reply to this Memorial has been discovered, and William Dick died on 4th April 1866.

With the charity of William Youatt at the time of the death of Edward Coleman, history might suggest that the Memorial was too close to Dick's last illness to secure a reply.

So be it.

In his own school and in his own country, Dick became a legend in his lifetime. The honest, hard-working, thrifty lad, sparing nothing of himself or his pocket for the good of his beloved profession. That legend has survived the grave, fostered by sister Mary, who long outlived him, and the Highland and Agricultural Society, and embalmed by merging Dick's name with the name of his school — the Royal (Dick) Veterinary College. His relentless opposition to the RCVS, from its birth to his death, and the true man, hide behind the legend. The former is readily discovered in the minutes of RCVS Council meetings, and elsewhere, but the man is blurred by a sycophantic veil. Clues to the truth are rare. Veterinary surgeon Rutherford recollecting instruction on pleuropneumonia from his student days: "We were taught by . . . the late Professor Dick, that the disease was not contagious. It was as much as our comfort at College was worth to question that opinion." Or veterinary surgeon Fleming, also recollecting his student days: "I never received five minutes' instruction in clinical medicine or practical knowledge . . . I had to trust to others and myself — *not* Professor Dick." Or, a codicil to Dick's will: "John Gamgee calling himself Principal and Professor of Veterinary Medicine in the New Veterinary College, Edinburgh, and his family and connections and the students or any of them who may have attended his classes or lectures, and shall be and are, each and all of them, hereby declared disqualified from acting as Professor, Lecturer or holding any situation whatever in or connected with the College as so founded by me."

In *The Veterinarian* for June 1866, Robert Bryden, veterinary surgeon of South Hetton, asked: "What is to be done with the holders of the diploma granted by the Highland and Agricultural Society? . . . I . . . humbly suggest . . . a petition" from the RCVS asking the Society "to withhold their diploma altogether . . . their consent will be all the more readily obtained now that Professor Dick is dead."

The RCVS continued to strive for a Veterinary Medical Bill, and in May 1866 it was agreed that it should be presented to Parliament. A month later, however, an anonymous pamphlet, "Reasons Why The Veterinary Surgeons' Bill Should Not Pass," was widely circulated. This originated in Edinburgh and forecast that the Bill would damage the Edinburgh veterinary school, making it subservient to "London," and

would devalue the Highland certificate. As a counter-measure, the proposition was resurrected, with powerful support from the Highland and
Agricultural Society, that there should be a separate veterinary charter
for Scotland.

Scots Members of Parliament McLaren and Leslie successfully blocked
the Bill, and all efforts to protect the title "veterinary surgeon" by a
Veterinary Medical Bill, all the meetings, all the discussions, deputations
and expense came to zero. The only compensation for the RCVS, after
many anxious months, was that a separate charter for Scotland was not
approved.

It would be misleading to infer that opposition to the RCVS from north
of Tweed was a perpetuation of Bannockburn and Flodden field. It was
not Scots v English, but the Edinburgh school and the Highland and
Agricultural Society v the RCVS. Many Scottish veterinary surgeons were
impressed by the existing corporate body's determination to improve the
status of the profession, and were opposed to the idea of a chartered
veterinary body in Scotland. Gamgee's achievement of affiliation of his
New Edinburgh school with the RCVS created a precedent. It was put to
good use by James McCall who founded a veterinary school in Glasgow in
1861. The RCVS Annual Report for 1865 recorded proudly: "Professor
McCall . . . has exhibited a wise discretion and soundness of judgement
in unhesitatingly affiliating his institution to the Royal College of Veterinary surgeons." McCall saw no need whatever for a Scottish charter.

*   *   *

George Bodington of Cardiff has a special place in British veterinary
history. He appears first as author of a letter to *The Veterinarian* for May
1862, entitled: "The Evil Of Empiricism As Connected With The Veterinary Profession." It is a forceful communication — belying its pon-
derous title — urging action against "*Quacks*" who call themselves
veterinary surgeons and "are daily examining horses as to soundness, and
have the effrontery to demand their half guinea fee, and write a certificate of their opinion." Bodington begs "every individual M.R.C.V.S.
to be '*up and doing*." *The Veterinarian* published many such cries for
action, but Bodington is distinguished by the fact that he practised as well
as preached.

In 1866 he asked the editors of *The Veterinarian* to announce that he
planned for the following year "a conference of the different veterinary
medical associations." The editors gave this initiative their "hearty

approval," and the first British Veterinary Congress was held in the Free-masons' Tavern, London, on Tuesday 7th May 1867. It was well attended and a great success.

John Lawson, President of the RCVS, took the chair at 9.0am, and after some preliminary comment, W. Litt of Shrewsbury gave a disserta-tion on that most vexed of equine topics: "The Law of Warranty." He was followed by Thomas Walton Mayer, of the Royal Engineers, Aldershot, prime architect of the 1844 Charter, who described: "The Charter· Its Objects." A contributor to the discussion expressed "gratitude to Mr Mayer for the manner in which he had given the entire history of the Charter. There were a great many who had not previously been aware of the details."

Mayer was followed by Professor Armatage of the Glasgow veterinary school with: "The Education Of The Veterinary Surgeon." This excellent paper stimulated vigorous discussion. Then Thomas Greaves of Man-chester on: "Provincial Veterinary Medical Associations; The Veterinary Mutual Defence And Benevolent Societies: Their Objects And Uses." Greaves traced the history of the Associations from the first in Manchester in 1851, to the tenth and most recent in the Midland Counties in 1866. He justly claimed that "these associations contain . . . the elements of great good and lasting benefit to our profession." Thomas Greaves did not believe in using one word if two could be pressed into service, but he was a great-hearted man, a worthy President of the RCVS in 1869, a philan-thropist in the Victorian manner, ready always to give time and money to professional brethren. His help to George Bodington was important for the success of this Congress.

It was accidental, but appropriate, that the last paper should be a final veterinary flourish from John Gamgee before his Albert school collapsed: "Epizootics, And How Influenced," a re-statement, with panache, of the veterinary significance of infectious diseases.

The 1867 Congress was a notable achievement, not repeated within a decade. It succeeded partly because it was well considered and well planned, but more because it was topical. The omens were good. The cloud to the north was lifting. The profession was uniting at last.

George Bodington? He served for a term on the RCVS Council, but he was an individualist not a committee man. He made this single unique contribution, and the editors of *The Veterinarian* kept faith with him. They published a detailed account of that historic day. A tale of able men looking to the future, determined, in the Bodington manner, to be up and doing.

CHAPTER 8

Preliminary and practical examinations — A new charter in 1876

It has been recorded that a paper on veterinary education at the Bodington Congress of 1867 stimulated vigorous discussion. It was presented by Professor George Armatage of the young veterinary school in Glasgow, and blew motes from many eyes. Armatage was dissatisfied with the "grovelling mediocrity" of the veterinary profession, largely to be explained, he declared, by inept selection of students and inadequate education.

He said: "I hold it to be indispensable that the veterinary surgeon should always be *the gentleman* . . . by education and training . . . our young men are occupied in warming and wearing down the seats of the class-room . . . theory in lieu of . . . solid practical application." Training was nominally for two years, but actually for two five-month sessions, with "no definite occupation during the summer vacation." Some "twenty-seven lectures per week" were packed into each session, with too little time for "dissections and clinical instruction." Only a short verbal examination separated ill-trained men from the coveted diploma.

He deplored a system that allowed "young men fresh from behind the anvil, the counter, or lawyer's desk, only half-furnished with the rudiments of their mother tongue . . . handwriting . . . sadly deficient, and diction exceedingly obscure" to enter a veterinary school, there to be exposed to a confusion of lectures they could not understand, and then after a perfunctory examination to be discharged as veterinary surgeons.

What were the remedies?

In summary, an examination before entering veterinary school to bar those who could not read and write English; a longer course to permit both practical and theoretical instruction; an examination that was practical as well as verbal.

Armatage ended with a plea for bursaries as "an improvement in the education of our students," and endowed lectureships to "stimulate the search for knowledge."

Opening the discussion, Mr Wilkinson supported the speaker, whose proposals would achieve "such respectability that ultimately . . . highly educated persons . . . would become veterinarians." Mr Smith agreed, and felt that "the rudiments of Latin and Greek" would not come amiss. Mr Greaves echoed the urgency for practical instruction. Mr Fleming put in a word for geology. Mr Ernes, a realist, thought a preliminary examination a good idea, but as the schools needed student fees in order to exist "he did not think the professors, hard working as they were, would do anything to counteract their interests." Messrs Naylor, Barnett, Wilson, Morgan, and many others, supported Armatage with gusto, and Mr Helmore was on his own in suggesting "that a man could be too highly educated in his profession." In short, there was overwhelming support for change — but the concept of bursaries and endowed lectureships fanciful beyond discussion.

Armatage proposed: "That the members of the Veterinary Congress desire to submit for the consideration of the principals of the veterinary colleges of Great Britain their sense of the necessity for an institution of the preliminary examination as a means of elevating the standing of the veterinary profession."

Mr Helmore, chastened by adverse comment, "begged to be allowed to second this resolution, lest it should be supposed he did not value education."

It was carried *nem. con.* .

Enthusiasm for educational improvement spread from the Congress to the country. The subject was debated by veterinary medical associations, with RCVS Councillors among their members, and reached the Council table within the year.

An editorial in *The Veterinarian* for June 1868 urged the RCVS to set a uniform standard of preliminary examination for all the schools, in accordance with "a common-sense interpretation of . . . the charter," for "it seems to us that the Council have absolute and unlimited power in respect to the institution of examinations."

Certainly the Council had the power, but they were not magicians to please all in a prickly population. With the Albert school dead, three schools remained — London, Edinburgh and Glasgow. All were private enterprises (albeit with differing executive constitutions), and each rivalled the others. The Scots were liable to close ranks against the English, but if English eyes were elsewhere Scot against Scot was fair fray. To harmonise all three in the matter of preliminary and practical examinations, the RCVS must balance an egg on the handle of a spoon.

In January 1869 they formed an "Examination Inquiry Committee."

This first reported to Council on 24th February. There was "very animated discussion," and general agreement that preliminary and practical examinations were essential. However, the Committee "expressed the great difficulty they had had . . . in consequence of the suggestions laid before them being somewhat indefinite in character." An echo, this, of the tribulations of any committee deputed to rationalise the opinions of Everyman.

It is to be noted that the London school had initiated a preliminary examination some five years previously, but Principal Spooner of that school now agreed to transfer responsibility for this examination from members of his staff to the independent College of Preceptors. He urged the RCVS to establish "a proper understanding" with "the respective teaching schools." There was relief within RCVS walls at this co-operation, for Charles Spooner was an autocratic, obstinate, unpredictable man.

Accepting Spooner's advice, an RCVS deputation led by President Greaves waited on the Governors of the London school on 13th July 1869, and was well received. The Chairman of the Governors "observed that we should all act together, and a representation should be made in writing to the other colleges." Letters were immediately sent by the RCVS to the Principals of the Edinburgh and Glasgow schools, asking each to meet a similar deputation. Glasgow agreed to a visit any time after mid-August, but Edinburgh could not find a spare hour in either August or September. The date eventually arranged for a conference in Scotland was 1st November 1869.

These dates emphasise the attitude of the schools to the RCVS at that time, and the manner in which the parent body had to tip-toe towards understanding with its children. Minutes of the RCVS Council meeting of 6th October 1869 at which the foray to the north was planned, read like preparations for a State visit to a hostile nation. All this pussy-footing just to ask the Scottish schools to join the London school in an examination embracing (1) writing for dictation (2) parsing a simple sentence (3) reading aloud (4) the first four rules of arithmetic and simple rule of three, to be carried out independently of both the veterinary schools and the RCVS.

Be it emphasised, however, that if unanimity *were* achieved it would be for the first time ever.

The presence of carefully selected Scottish graduates in the RCVS deputation to Scotland no doubt contributed to the goodwill with which

it was received. Certainly the visitors "had much reason for being gratified with the frank and unhesitating manner" in which the Scots "signified their approval of and adhesion to the great principle to which the
Royal College of Veterinary Surgeons was endeavouring to give practical
effect."

An immediate answer to a simple question was impossible, of course,
for the proposal had to be "put into such form" as could be examined
more closely. This occupied several months, and maintained the proper
distance between Edinburgh and London.

In the event, general acceptance of a preliminary examination for all
students aspiring to enter a veterinary school was reported to the profession at the Annual General Meeting in 1870. The standard would be
uniform between the schools. It had been hoped that there would be independent examiners; the College of Preceptors in London, and the
Rectors of the High Schools of Edinburgh and Glasgow in those cities,
respectively. At the last moment, however, Principal McCall of Glasgow
"resiled from that agreement" and "persisted in examining intending
students himself."

The precedent of unanimity between the RCVS and the schools had
again eluded capture.

A practical examination was achieved in 1871. Its stilted evolution
resembled that of the preliminary examination, with the difference that
this time there was discord in London with the Scottish schools in harmony. Disagreement was over location of the examination. The Scots
were willing to provide animals — lame horses and the like — in or near
their own premises, but Principal Charles Spooner refused to provide
facilities within the London school. Indeed, at a meeting of the RCVS
Council in November 1870 he tried to kill the idea of a practical examination altogether. He said: "If you think that you are going to put the screw
upon us by instituting what I should call a fanciful, imperfect examination . . . you are very much mistaken." In mitigation of this outburst, it
may be noted that at this time Spooner was showing signs of mental
aberration, and he died some twelve months later. He lived long enough,
however, to force the RCVS to seek help from the Markets Committee of
the Corporation of London, who "gratuitously placed the extensive
cattle lairs and market area at Islington at the disposal of the Council."

The RCVS practical examination for graduating students was fully
organised by 1872. In London it was held at the Cattle Market, Islington,
and in Mr Matthew's cab-yard in Theobald's Road. In Glasgow the venue
was Principal McCall's own farm. In Edinburgh horses were examined in
the College yard, and cattle in a market near the school. In August 1872,

after Spooner's death, the Governors of the London school, briefed by the new Principal James Beart Simonds, invited the RCVS "to conduct the practical examination of the pupils of this College in the Institution."

Achievement of preliminary and practical examinations was a milestone in the progress of the RCVS to *de facto* leadership of the profession. Wise counsel from the Country (interpreted by George Armatage at the 1867 Congress) had been heeded. Patient diplomacy had won co-operation from sensitive schools. A properly educated profession was in sight. Above all, the demoralising years of kicks and butts were past.

*　　*　　*

The Edinburgh school was reorganised after the death of William Dick in 1866. Dick, a bachelor, made ample provision for Mary his unmarried sister, but bequeathed his school to the city of Edinburgh, the Lord Provost and Town Council to be trustees. J.H.B. Hallen, of Her Majesty's Bombay Army, joined the three other members of staff as Principal. Hallen was recalled to India within a year, however, and was replaced in 1867 by William Williams, veterinary surgeon of Bradford. Williams had entered Dick's school as a student on returning from a do-or-die — but wholly successful — trip to Australia to fight pulmonary tuberculosis with hard work and sunshine. All went well for a time, but increasing friction between Williams and the school's trustees led to his resignation in 1873. He immediately established a veterinary school of his own in the city, and four-fifths of the students left Clyde Street to join him in Gayfield Square. His New Edinburgh school was affiliated by Sign Manual to the RCVS in 1874, and was the second school so named. The first New Edinburgh school was that of John Gamgee, founded in 1857 and removed to London as the Albert school in 1865.

William Fearnley of Leeds followed Williams at the Edinburgh school, but he too could not work with the trustees and was replaced in 1874 by Thomas Walley, already on the staff. Walley's Principalship, to his death in 1894, was a progressive period during which the school grew in stature and prestige.

There was an important change at the London school, too, when Simonds became Principal after the death of Charles Spooner in 1871. Simonds has already been mentioned as first Professor of Cattle Pathology at the London school in 1842, as a signatory of the 1844 Charter, as recognising the exotic diseases sheep-pox in 1847 and cattle plague in 1865, and as first veterinary surgeon in the veterinary department created by the Privy Council to deal with cattle plague. On becoming Principal he gave up his part-time duties in the Privy Council office (to be succeeded by G.T. Brown), and concentrated his considerable administrative and scientific abilities on improving every aspect of the school, for which he obtained a Charter of Incorporation in 1875.

*   *   *

It is clear from *The Veterinarian*, that practising veterinary surgeons of the mid-nineteenth century diagnosed disease exactly as did their forefathers. Cases were assessed by eye, ear, nose and touch. Hot head. Cold feet. Tight skin. Dry tongue. The most skilful men were those who had seen most and remembered most. This was the veterinary Art; tolerably successful, in spite of little understanding. Anatomy stood higher than physiology in performance of the Art.

As the century progressed, however, Art was threatened by Science. Estimation gave way to measurement, and mechanical aids revolutionised veterinary diagnosis. One of the first and most useful was the clinical thermometer.

It has been mentioned that in 1865, at the Albert veterinary school in London, John Gamgee measured the body temperature of animals in the incubative and clinical stages of cattle plague, and concluded that a rise in temperature was associated with the disease. This was the first veterinary application of the clinical thermometer in Britain. Its usefulness in human medicine had lately been recognised, but the novelty of the procedure may be gauged from the fact that at a meeting of the RCVS Council in July 1866, Gamgee "begged to present to the Museum two registering thermometers made by Mr Cassella."

By 1869 George Armatage (the same who had spoken on veterinary education at the 1867 Congress) was able to present a considerable amount of original information in a pamphlet: "The Thermometer as an Aid to Diagnosis in Veterinary Medicine." He gave credit to "Mr L. Cassella, Philosophical Instrument Maker to the Admiralty, of Hatton Garden, London, for the perfection to which the clinical thermometer has been raised," and provided proof of the diagnostic significance of variations in the rectal temperature in animals. He emphasised "the infallible test of approaching contagious disease, its gradual progress in intensity, or the more welcome approach of convalescence." His readers were in no doubt that the clinical thermometer had come to stay.

*   *   *

Genial, generous, W.J.T. Morton died in 1868. His unique distinction was as first recipient of the RCVS diploma in 1844. His working life was at the London school, from clerk and dispenser in 1822 to retirement as

Professor of Chemistry in 1860. Ill-health prevented his acceptance of the RCVS Presidency in 1867. His co-editorship with Simonds of *The Veterinarian* after Percivall's death in 1854 was vital for the profession. It is believed to have been Morton who chose for the London Veterinary Medical Association of 1836 the motto *Vis unita fortior*, later adopted by the RCVS.

Another link with the earliest RCVS days was lost in the following year when William Joseph Goodwin died. His signature was on the Charter, for which he and his father had worked valiantly. Goodwin was veterinary surgeon to George IV, William IV and Queen Victoria. He was President of the RCVS in 1853, and was the driving force in acquiring in that year its first permanent home at No 10 Red Lion Square.

*   *   *

"They have their exits and their entrances."

Morton and Goodwin to the wings.

Fleming and Fitzwygram to the centre of the stage.

Forge-boy George Fleming, born in Glasgow in 1833, son of a farrier, so impressed his employer, veterinary surgeon John Lawson of Manchester, that Lawson enrolled him in the Edinburgh veterinary school. He won medals and obtained the Highland certificate in 1855, then joined the Army. He served in the Crimea, China, Syria and Egypt before settling in England. Industrious beyond belief, a compulsive writer of letters, essays, articles and books, linguist and translator, organiser and politician, he revelled in RCVS affairs. In 1866 he added the MRCVS diploma to his Highland certificate, and was elected to the RCVS Council two years later. He was deeply involved in negotiating the RCVS preliminary and practical examinations. Ambition drove him without mercy, and shortened his temper. He was briefly associated with *The Veterinarian*, but craved a personal audience. In 1875 he founded *The Veterinary Journal*, saying editorially, "For a number of years, the great majority, if not all, of the members of the Veterinary profession have felt that neither their views nor their interests have been adequately or fairly represented, owing to the absence of an independent journal . . ."

When Fleming drew his talents, modesty was missed.

Bombast apart, *The Veterinary Journal* was a first-class scientific, educational and political monthly.

Frederick Wellington John Fitzwygram was ten years older than Fleming. Ultimately a fourth baronet, he was educated at Eton and Sandhurst, and was only vaguely aware of the world of toil. He was commissioned in the 6th Dragoons in July 1843, and seemed destined for pigsticking and intellectual oblivion. In his thirties, however, to his utmost credit and to the good fortune of the veterinary profession, he attended the Edinburgh veterinary school, in amateur fashion, to broaden his interest in horses. Stimulated by the lectures, he continued this unpremeditated education, and in 1854 — accidentally, as it were — acquired the Highland certificate and became a veterinary surgeon. Service overseas prevented intimate contact with the profession until the 1870's, when he was finally stationed in England. In 1871 he added the MRCVS diploma to his Edinburgh certificate (as Fleming had already done). In 1872 he was elected a Vice-President (an ex-officio member of Council), in 1873 a Councillor, and in 1875 President of the RCVS.

This crash course to stardom was partly unearned, in that in those days an aristocrat had ten lengths start over a pleb in any race, and partly due to exceptional administrative ability. By 1875 Fitzwygram had had many years in senior management; in particular, he was an outstandingly competent chairman. His high social status was crucially important to the veterinary profession, for he could face anyone on equal terms, including the titled gentlemen of Scotland's Highland and Agricultural Society.

The complementary talents of Fleming and Fitzwygram made veterinary history in 1876, and for several years thereafter.

On 14th July 1875 at the first RCVS Council meeting after his election as President, everyone was impressed by Fitzwygram's brisk style of chairmanship and interest in education. He drove straight into the RCVS/schools minefield, and launched a revolution.

By the next meeting in October, his ideas had crystallized into a proposal for an extended Charter. He suggested that this should cover election of Council by voting papers, a registration fee for all members of the profession, a higher degree, RCVS meetings elsewhere than in London, extended powers to deal with professional misconduct, special regulations for medical men wishing to become veterinary surgeons, professors to be examiners, protection of the designation 'veterinary surgeon.'

He moved that it was "desirable to apply for an extended Charter."

Fleming seconded the motion, which he had obviously discussed with Fitzwygram beforehand. He was emphatic that the profession required a higher degree. The motion was carried, and a committee was appointed to "take the matter into consideration and report."

Fitzwygram's stand on education was unequivocal. Within a few days of this Council meeting, he told the distinguished audience at the inaugural meeting of the London veterinary school's autumn session, that he "trusted that the day was near at hand when none but thoroughly educated students would be permitted to enter the ranks of the profession."

It might be considered tactless to have commented thus in that seat of learning, but it was a message that even the doorman understood.

With two Army men in the driving seat, the committee had to report at the double. Even the Council's Parliamentary agent W.A. Loch was shocked into immediate action. In a letter dated 18th November 1875 he wrote: "I now send you Draft Supplemental Charter for the Royal College of Veterinary Surgeons. Its terms will of course demand much consideration . . ." He had misjudged Fitzwygram, who, although prepared to listen briefly to suggested amendments, urgently required a definitive document. The Draft was reproduced for public scrutiny in *The Veterinarian* in January 1876.

The first paragraph caused controversy: "From henceforth the corporate name or style of the . . . body politic and corporate shall be 'The Royal Veterinary University.' "

This suggestion may seem pretentious, but the reason was the practical one that there was (and, indeed, still is) irritating confusion between 'The Royal Veterinary College,' the teaching school at Camden Town, and 'The Royal College of Veterinary Surgeons,' the administrators of the corporate body.

The intention was good, but *The British Medical Journal* commented: "An university with the sole function of conferring diplomas or degrees on veterinary surgeons would be a strange anomaly," and *The Lancet* hoped: "That the council of the college will perceive in time that such a change of title would cover them with ridicule." Six months later, giving their verdict on the Charter application, their Lordships of the Privy Council agreed with the medical press, and could not "advise Her Majesty to sanction the adoption . . . of the proposed title of 'University.' " However, they were "prepared to recommend Her Majesty's approval" of the other clauses. These covered election of Fellows, election of Honorary and Foreign Associates, use of voting papers, location of the Annual General Meeting, removal of names from the Register, appointment of a Registrar, maintenance of a Register, appointment of Secretary, and power to hold land.

The regretted omission was control of unlicensed practice. This had been an important original objective, but, as Fitzwygram had to explain to a disappointed Annual General Meeting, it had become clear that "a prohibitory clause such as was desired could only be obtained by an Act of Parliament."

The 1876 Charter was a remarkable twelve-month achievement for Fitzwygram, with Fleming dominant in the Council. It was no wonder that Fitzwygram was elected President for a second term, and no wonder that Fitzwygram nominated Fleming for re-election to the Council, an election in which he easily topped the poll.

Fitzwygram and Fleming had the profession in their hands.

Charter now. Act later.

CHAPTER 9

The Highland Certificate abandoned — Veterinary Surgeons Act 1881

The consequences of a discovery reported in 1876 were enormous. German physician Robert Koch published proof that Casimir Davaine's microscopic Bacteria were the cause of anthrax. He supplied the clues that had eluded Davaine, the excitement of whose researches, it will be recalled, had been captured by *The Veterinarian* in 1864. The mystery of infectious disease was solved. The concept of spontaneous generation was dead. Dead, that is, in a historical sense, because there continued for several years to be disbelievers in a germ theory of disease, eminent men among them. For example, Henry Charlton Bastian, MD, FRS, of University College Hospital, London, whose criticism of Koch and poohpoohing of Pasteur make him the most mistaken pedant in the history of biology.

The technical wizardry of Koch's first paper will never be surpassed. In a series of meticulous observations on the anthrax bacillus, he established the credibility of medical bacteriology. Veterinarians had special interest in the work, because, although occurring occasionally in man, anthrax is intrinsically a disease of animals.

In essence, Koch's achievement was two-fold. First, he demonstrated that the anthrax bacillus could exist not only in the rod-shaped form seen by Davaine in the blood of animals that had died of the disease, but also in a highly resistant resting form, or spore, that changed to the active disease-producing rod under favourable conditions. Thus was explained the haphazard occurrence of clinical disease, hitherto attributed to spontaneous generation. Secondly, he proved that only the anthrax bacillus produced anthrax.

These discoveries, so simple in summary, were born of months of patient observation. Koch was a medical practitioner in the small town of Wollstein, and study of anthrax was in spare time with home-made apparatus. In April 1876 he explained his findings to Ferdinand Cohn,

Professor of Botany in Breslau. Their importance was immediately recognised, and Koch was encouraged to develop his researches.

Within a year Louis Pasteur and his colleague Jules Joubert had confirmed Koch's observations, and the stage was set for an exciting era in the understanding of infectious diseases. The British veterinary profession, with *The Veterinarian* (still edited by Simonds) leading, began to grasp the meaning of these new ideas. Not everyone immediately, of course. Indeed, in 1877 the impetuous William Williams, Principal of the New Edinburgh school, missed the epidemiological significance of the anthrax spore when he summarised Koch's work for the Yorkshire Veterinary Medical Society. He said: "We can arrive at but one conclusion . . . one disease contagious by inoculation . . . has been clearly traced to . . . other causes than infection, that, in fact, it originates spontaneously . . . How some writers have concluded so positively that contagious diseases cannot *now* arise spontaneously is beyond my comprehension."

Which comment makes the more remarkable the refusal twelve years earlier of Simonds and Gamgee to accept a spontaneous origin for cattle plague and other infectious diseases.

*　　*　　*

Several clauses in the supplemental Charter of 1876 dealt with a new breed — Fellows of the RCVS. The Council was instructed "before the expiration of six calendar months from the date hereof, and in such manner as the Council shall deem best," to elect as Primary Fellows, without examination, men with at least fifteen years professional experience and a claim to distinction. Thereafter, election to Fellowship would be by examination.

Invidious choice!

A Fellowship Committee tried to be impartial by listing qualifications that would attract Fellowship status: previous Presidents of the RCVS, Professors, Examiners, the Father of the Profession. These were easily identified, but who were "Veterinary Authors"? Would publication of a few letters qualify? An article, a pamphlet, or must it be a book? Who had shown "Distinction in Original Research"? By whom assessed? The irritant above all, however, was the requirement that Primary Fellows "shall have practised as veterinary surgeons for fifteen years at least." Did this mean that they must have been Members of the RCVS for fifteen years? Or might men with the Highland certificate for fifteen years and the MRCVS diploma for a shorter time (of whom there were many) also qualify?

Oh, recipe for squabble! If the Highlanders were ineligible, Fitz-wygram and Fleming, originators of the Fellowship idea, would be excluded.

At the RCVS Council meeting of 11th January 1877: "The President said the following letter had been received from Mr Greaves . . ." This was Thomas Greaves, benevolent, generous-in-spirit-and-in-pocket former President of the RCVS. His letter dated 5th January began: "I intended if I had been present to raise the question of opening the door a little wider for the admission of Fellows . . . we are excluding many of our best men." It ended by proposing that "those gentlemen who have . . . gained the Highland Society's Certificate fifteen years ago . . . and are now holders of our Diploma, shall be deemed eligible to be elected Fellows."

Is it improper to wonder if the felicitous timing of this letter was accidental? Certainly President Fitzwygram converted it immediately into a formal motion, seconded by Thomas Greaves (fortuitously present after all), and "carried, Professor Simonds dissenting."

Simonds dissented because two years previously Her Majesty had gra-ciously agreed to a Charter of Incorporation of the Royal Veterinary College (the London teaching school), of which Simonds was Principal, that included provision for "appointing former students of the College, *Licentiates*, or those who have practised with particular distinction . . . *Fellows*." Not surprisingly, he viewed the push by Fitzwygram and Flem-ing for Fellows of the Royal College of Veterinary Surgeons (the corporate body) as plagiarism. Which indeed it was, although with goodwill the two might have co-existed. However, Fleming was furious when the school obtained a Charter (although it did not affect the RCVS), and he was rude to Simonds in an editorial in the November 1875 number of the recently established *Veterinary Journal*.

In consequence, Simonds and those members of his staff who had been invited to become RCVS Fellows declined the honour. They were not alone. Of the invitations issued, seventy-seven were accepted (including Fitzwygram and Fleming), and sixteen were refused. Some feathers were ruffled by the invitation, others by its absence.

All in all, a profitless plunge into deep waters.

But there was an illuminating sequel.

On 1st May 1877 President Fitzwygram showed the RCVS Council the mettle of his leadership. A letter dated 19th April 1877 from the Lord President of the Council had been dealt with personally by Fitzwygram. It was an important letter, informing the RCVS that the London school had applied for a supplemental Charter, of which a copy was enclosed, and asking for observations.

Fitzwygram now explained that under the old Charter of the London school "the Governors could only be elected from among the subscribers, and no veterinary surgeon was permitted to be a subscriber. The object of the supplemental Charter was to allow veterinary surgeons to be placed on the Board."

Then the gritty bit.

Fitzwygram further explained that the London school "of their own good feeling had also taken measures to cancel the power they had obtained to create Fellows, as it was thought that that degree would interfere with the . . . rights of the Royal College of Veterinary Surgeons."

Secretary Coates was bidden to read a reply (formulated by Fitzwygram) to the Privy Council, sent by return of post:-

"20th April 1877

Sir,

I have the honour to acknowledge the receipt of your letter of the 19th inst., with the draft supplemental Charter prayed for by the Royal Veterinary College enclosed therein, and in reply I am directed by the President and Council of the Royal College of Veterinary Surgeons to say that the draft of the proposed supplemental Charter meets with their entire approbation, and that they have consequently no observations to make therein."

Fitzwygram then said "that the letter had been sent before obtaining the approval of the Council, but he presumed it expressed the general feeling. He apologised to the Council for the mistake which had been made in sending it before their approval had been obtained."

There is no record of comment from the Council. It could be that they were literally dumbfounded.

Has any other RCVS President informed the Privy Council, in writing, that a matter has met with "entire approbation," when it has been neither raised nor discussed?

In explanation, this autocracy was a means justified by an objective. Fitzwygram was determined to raise for ever the portcullis that barred professional progress — the Highland certificate still being granted at the Edinburgh veterinary school.

Fitzwygram knew the personalities within the profession, and their prejudices. His unique position as aristocrat with a large private income, veterinary surgeon (holder of both the Highland certificate and the diploma of the RCVS), President of the RCVS (re-elected in 1877 for a third consecutive year), and a Governor of the London school, enabled him to ignore 'the usual channels.' He knew that to have Fellows of the London school and Fellows of the RCVS would end in rivalry. Although the former had precedence, the latter were more professionally relevant, so he had quietly persuaded the Governors of the London school to abandon the idea, and had given the RCVS Council no opportunity to discuss the matter. That Simonds had had to forfeit his brain-child was less important than that the Highland Society should have one less cause for complaint.

Active advance against the Highland citadel dates from a well attended meeting of the Liverpool Veterinary Medical Association on 12th July 1877. *The Veterinarian's* account of that meeting begins: "Mr. G. Fleming . . . introduced the question of the desirability of obtaining an Act of Parliament . . . protective to the interests of the profession . . . Sir F. Fitzwygram . . . said the real question was whether it was judicious to apply at the present time for an Act . . . one great obstacle . . . was the . . . diploma of the Highland and Agricultural Society . . . they should endeavour to induce by argument and not by pressure the . . . Society to withdraw their examination . . . Mr Greaves . . . also thought it would be unwise to go for an Act of Parliament in the present state of feeling."

Then, at a meeting of the RCVS Council on 2nd January 1878 President Fitzwygram proposed that holders of the Highland certificate be awarded the MRCVS diploma after examination and payment of a fee. His elaboration of the proposal was shrewd and fair, and provoked mature discussion. There was strong support from Greaves, Fleming and others, and positive quest for reconciliation of attitudes and interests. Finally, Fitzwygram "had no hesitation in assenting to . . . postponement of the debate, because it was a question which required much consideration."

For the next few months *the* veterinary talking point was an accommodation between the Highland Society and the RCVS, so that by 6th May an RCVS Annual General Meeting was prepared for, and approved, Fitzwygram's motion that power be "given to the Council to appoint a committee to confer with the Highland and Agricultural Society in regard to the discontinuance of their examination."

The pace now quickened.

On 4th June Fitzwygram agreed to an extension of his RCVS Presidency for a fourth year, because "it had been represented to him that with regard to the abolition of the Highland and Agricultural Society's certificate, he might be, for various reasons, an acceptable negotiator . . . he owed what he possessed, in regard to veterinary matters, to the school of Professor Dick, which was now more or less represented by the Highland and Agricultural Society. This would induce him to go into the pending negotiations in a kind and friendly manner."

Everyone sighed thankfully, for they knew that not only was Fitzwygram an acceptable negotiator, but that he was the *only* ambassador likely to succeed. There would be a negotiating committee of three: Fitzwygram, James Collins, Principal Veterinary Surgeon of the Army, and William Robertson, practitioner of Kelso.

A month later Fitzwygram reported to the RCVS Council that "he had met the Secretary of the Highland and Agricultural Society about a fortnight ago in Paris, and had subsequently . . . had a conversation with him in London." The negotiating committee had received from the Society a statement of the conditions on which they would end their Edinburgh examination. Of these, the most important was that their certificate holders must be given the RCVS diploma without examination. The negotiating committee recommended acceptance of this condition, because "the scheme would be an entire failure" unless "liberal terms" were offered. The other conditions were negotiable, and Council agreed to discuss them further with the Society.

A draft agreement between the RCVS and the Society was slightly amended by the RCVS Council on 2nd October, and a final agreement was approved on 15th January 1879. Application was then made to the Privy Council for a supplementary Charter. This was approved seven months later. No new applicant for the Highland certificate was accepted after 1st January 1879.

It was a notable performance. By patience, guile, administrative acumen and commonsense, Fitzwygram had given new life to the veterinary profession. Was ever a more acceptable man in a more appropriate place at a more critical moment? No one else could have unified a profession torn so unhappily asunder. The benefit of his wisdom is beyond reckoning, and those who pass his life-size portrait at the Royal College of Veterinary Surgeons should genuflect in gratitude.

The RCVS was now master of its destiny, but an Act of Parliament was required to ensure that holders of its diploma were the only veterinary surgeons recognised in law.

In May 1879 William Williams, Principal of the New Edinburgh school, succeeded Fitzwygram as RCVS President. He was less interested in an Act than some of his Council colleagues would have wished. George Fleming, in particular, craved action. In January 1880 he could wait no longer, and gave notice to the Council that at the next quarterly meeting he would move: "That steps be immediately taken by the Royal College of

Veterinary Surgeons to obtain an Act of Parliament for the protection of the title of 'Veterinary Surgeon,' or other titles conferred by Royal Charter." The motion was approved in April 1880, having been seconded by Principal Thomas Walley of the Edinburgh (Dick's) veterinary school.

On 25th May Fleming succeeded Williams as RCVS President, and acquired freedom to urge immediate plans to obtain an Act. He was supported by the ever-helpful Thomas Greaves, who emphasised that the road had been cleared by removal of "the difficulty of the Highland Society." Greaves asked, however, what the possible cost might be. In reply, Fleming said that "he could form no estimate." The proposition to seek an Act was passed to the Parliamentary Committee of the Council for early report.

That report did not materialise, for the reason that discussions outside the Council chamber brought the proposed Veterinary Medical Act to the attention of the Royal Society for the Prevention of Cruelty to Animals (RSPCA). The Society was interested because if the title 'veterinary surgeon' were protected, the general public would be able to distinguish between trained veterinary surgeons and quacks, and medical and surgical treatment of animals would in consequence improve. In private discussion, Fleming was so persuasive that Earl Spencer, Lord President of the Privy Council, agreed to take charge of the Bill, making it a Government measure, and Lord Aberdare, President of the RSPCA, promised to introduce it to the Lords.

Fleming explained this to the RCVS Council in December 1880, and added that "the draft of the Bill has been prepared by an eminent parliamentary draughtsman."

This was miraculous support. However, some doubt was expressed by Councillors Greaves and Harpley (the latter an ex-President of the RCVS with special knowledge of Parliamentary procedure) that the title 'veterinary surgeon' could thus be restricted to holders of the RCVS diploma. Both believed that some degree of recognition would have to be given to unqualified men who had been earning their living as 'veterinary surgeons.'

How right they were!

The draft Bill published in *The Veterinary Journal* for February 1881 made it an offence for anyone not holding the RCVS diploma to "wilfully and falsely pretend to be or take or use the title of Veterinary Surgeon." As predicted by Greaves and Harpley, this was rejected by the legal advisers to the Crown, because the 1844 Charter conferred only privileges, and anyone might call himself a veterinary surgeon without breaking the law. In that form the Bill would certainly be rejected.

Restraint on use of the title 'veterinary surgeon' could only be prospective.

The Lord President of the Privy Council and Lord Aberdare were so impressed by the need for legislation, however, that they had the Bill amended and its scope extended. The revised version was published in *The Veterinary Journal* for May 1881, with the comment that it "is greatly improved in shape, and made more complete in several important particulars, and . . . the designation has been altered from 'Veterinary Medical Bill' to 'Veterinary Surgeons' Bill.' "

Other amendments followed, so that by July *The Veterinary Journal* concluded that if all were eventually included "the Bill . . . will be of a far more important character than before, and place the profession . . . on quite an equal footing with the medical profession." The Bill had indeed changed dramatically in six months. Unqualified men styling themselves veterinary surgeons had created such a rumpus that "the Lord President and Lord Aberdare could not resist their claim." Prominent among the unqualified men demanding inclusion in any new definition of 'veterinary surgeon,' were the small number of Highland certificate holders who had refused to pay the modest fee required under the 1879 Charter to acquire the RCVS diploma. For this reason, the Highland and Agricultural Society opposed the Bill. As Fleming remarked tartly, via *The Veterinary Journal*: "Any attempt to improve the position of the profession appears to act upon a small section in Edinburgh as a red rag is said to do upon a bull."

Time was running out. There was a nail-biting finish to the bid for an Act. If the Bill were not passed that session, momentum would be lost and there would be stouter opposition from those already digging trenches.

Lord Spencer saw the Bill through the Lords. Opposition from the Lord Chancellor caused loss of the clause exempting veterinary surgeons from jury service, but that was a luxury extra and the main clauses survived. At Lord Spencer's request, the Vice-President of the Privy Council, the Right Honourable W.J. Mundella, took charge in the Commons to ensure that the Bill was not lost in the press of end-of-session business. He dealt skilfully with opposition to the clauses concerning unqualified practitioners, and with an out-of-the-blue objection (historically inexplicable) by Messrs Morgan, Reynolds and Taylor of the RCVS Council, who suddenly declared the Bill futile and unnecessary. This latter objection startled the good Mundella, for he had been assured of unanimous support within the RCVS. It almost holed the ship.

To abbreviate: the Bill received the Royal Assent on 27th August 1881, as the Members were rising for the summer recess.

The provisions of this momentous Act were summarised in the RCVS report for 1881 – 82. There were eighteen clauses:-

"The Register of Veterinary Surgeons is to be received as evidence in courts of law and elsewhere, and the functions of the Registrar are defined with regard to the admission and removal of names from the Register. The circumstances under which names may be removed are also defined, and the legal responsibility for removal is assumed by the Privy Council. Penalties are imposed for obtaining registration by false representation, and provision made for the registration of colonial or foreign practitioners with recognised diplomas, under certain conditions. The Charters, present and future, of the Royal College, are made statutory and are confirmed by the Act. Unqualified practitioners who had continuously practised Veterinary Medicine and Surgery for five years previous to the passing of the Act are to claim registration, and the names of those whose claim is admitted by the Council of the Royal College are to be entered in a separate register under the heading Existing Practitioner. This registration confers no privileges whatever, or acknowledgement that these persons are anything more than unqualified practitioners, and merely protects them from the penal operations of the Act. They are in no way to be considered as Members of the Royal College; and after the passing of the Act, neither they nor other persons can take or use any name, title, addition or description by means of initials or letters placed after their names or otherwise, stating or implying that they are Fellows or Members of the Royal College, without incurring penalty.

This provision will enable the Royal College to register only those whom it considers have been practising Veterinary Medicine and Surgery continuously for five years previous to August 27th, 1876, and who are of certified good moral character; and also at once to institute proceedings against those who falsely represent themselves as Fellows or Members of the Royal College, or in any respect as legally qualified practitioners. After December 31st, 1883, no unregistered person, or one who does not hold the Veterinary Certificate of the Highland and Agricultural Society, can take or use any name, title, addition or description implying that he practises Veterinary Surgery or any branch thereof, without being liable to punishment; nor can such person recover payment for performing an operation, giving Veterinary attendance or advice, or acting in any way as a Veterinary Surgeon or practitioner."

The Report gave special thanks to Lord Aberdare and the RSPCA, to

Earl Spencer, to Mr Mundella, and to Colonel Kingscote, M.P.. George Fleming, too, was thanked — and everybody knew that it was he who had borne the fiery heat and burdens of those days.

Who paid for the Act? The truth was so little publicised at the time, that later speculation suggested the RSPCA as Fairy Godmother. Not so. The story is in the minutes of the RCVS Council meeting for 4th October 1881. The President, George Fleming, paid all expenses out of his own pocket. He "believed the Act had not cost the Royal College of Veterinary Surgeons one penny, and it was not his wish or intention that it should." The minutes continue: "After some conversation, in which some of the members endeavoured to persuade the President to have the expenses refunded, the President said he felt it would be a slight on him if the matter were not allowed to remain as it stood. It was then, in deference to the wishes of the President, allowed to drop."

Fitzwygram the Charter. Fleming the Act. Strides that emancipated the profession from the serfdom of internal strife. Arguments on ways and means there would always be, but never again numbing sectarianism to kill the consensus of democracy.

CHAPTER 10

A national veterinary association

Two bacteriological discoveries announced at the London International Medical Congress of 1881, affected every human being and every domesticated animal in the world.

One by Robert Koch, the other by Louis Pasteur.

Koch explained how to obtain micro-organisms in pure culture. He demonstrated the technique in the Physiological Laboratory of King's College, London, to Joseph Lister (initiator of antiseptic surgery), John Burdon Sanderson (Professor of Physiology, University College, London), Jean Chauveau (French veterinary anatomist and bacteriologist), and Louis Pasteur.

A 'pure culture' is a growth of a single species of micro-organism in a nutrient medium. A 'nutrient medium' is a concoction, such as meat broth, that contains the food required by a micro-organism. If there is more than one species of micro-organism in a culture it is described as 'contaminated.' By trial and error, early bacteriologists had prepared liquid media to suit the needs of a host of different micro-organisms. Many people guessed that certain organisms caused certain diseases. But which caused which? Koch had established for anthrax the principle of one-organism-one-disease, but micro-organisms are ubiquitous and it was so difficult to obtain, and to maintain, pure cultures that there had been little further progress for five frustrating years.

Now Koch had the answer.

From earlier published observations on the growth of micro-organisms on *solid* — as distinct from in *liquid* — media, he surmised that if a single unit (a cell) of a micro-organism settled on a solid nutrient medium, it would grow into a blob (a colony) exclusively of that organism. The guess was correct. With unique technical virtuosity, he experimented with various solid media, and found that warmed meat extract mixed with gelatine could be cooled to a solid, transparent pabulum. When the tip of a needle previously sterilised by heat, was dipped into a contaminated *liquid* culture and then drawn across this *solid* medium, colonies appeared a few days later along the needle-track. Those of the same colour, shape and size were of the same micro-organism, and differed from colonies of other organisms. Colonies of each organism could then be picked off with a sterilised needle, each to begin a pure culture in a liquid medium.

An eye-witness of this miraculous demonstration recorded that Pasteur said to Koch: "C'est un grand progrès, Monsieur!"

Within a year Koch had identified the tubercle bacillus by this new technique, and Loeffler and Schutz the organism of glanders. In 1884 Koch isolated the organism of Asiatic cholera, Loeffler the diphtheria bacillus, Gaffky the typhoid bacillus. Then, in breath-taking succession, staphylococcus, streptococcus, gonococcus, pneumococcus, mening-ococcus, the tetanus bacillus . . . almost *ad infinitum*.

Pasteur's discovery was of attenuation of micro-organisms, key to a new science — immunology. There are optimal conditions for growth of all living things: heat, humidity, light and so on. Pasteur discovered that sub-optimal conditions not only affected the growth of micro-organisms, but were liable also to reduce their propensity to cause disease. This he called 'attenuation.' While studying fowl cholera, a highly lethal disease of chickens, he noticed that injection of young cultures of the causal organism killed many birds, but that old cultures were far less deadly. Others might have thus observed, but it was Pasteur's talent to wonder why, and his genius to guess that a first injection of old (attenuated) culture would protect against a second of full virulence. He had confirmed experimentally what Jenner had found empirically; that resistance to disease (immunity) can be artificially produced. Indeed, Pasteur was so conscious of his intellectual debt to Jenner, that, at the London Medical Congress of 1881, he suggested that "au mérite et aux immenses services rendus par un des plus grands hommes de l'Angleterre, votre Jenner," the terms 'vaccine' and 'vaccination' should not be limited to smallpox, but should apply to artificial immunisation against all diseases. A proposal accepted without dissent.

Pasteur extended the principle of attenuation to the anthrax bacillus, and in 1881 at Pouilly-le-Fort carried out a successful vaccination experiment with sheep and cattle, the story of which was sent round an astonished world by M. de Blowitz, Paris correspondent of *The Times* of London. No wonder that at the London congress a few months later Pasteur mistook his rapturous reception for acclamation at the arrival of the Prince of Wales. "But it is you that they are all cheering," his colleagues said. He was immortalised in 1885 when his immunological skill saved from death little Joseph Meister of Alsace, torn in hands and legs by a rabid dog. The first of thousands thus reprieved.

Pasteur's researches revolutionised medical and veterinary attitudes throughout the world. He encouraged veterinary science in Britain, and in 1882 became an Honorary Associate of the RCVS. In 1886 he welcomed to his laboratory in Paris Professors Robertson and Penberthy of the London veterinary school, whose visit was financed by the Royal Agricultural Society of England. For some two weeks the visitors were instructed by Pasteur's colleagues Charles Chamberland and Émile Roux in "the method there adopted for the preparation of vaccines."

The Professor Robertson who visited Pasteur's laboratory in 1886, was William Robertson, one-time practitioner in Kelso, who in 1881 succeeded Simonds as Principal of the London veterinary school. Simonds, at seventy-one, feeling the strain of a mentally and physically demanding life, had asked the Governors to relieve him of lecturing duties. They readily agreed, but at the same time indicated that he had reached an age at which he should retire. Autobiographically he wrote: "This suggestion I was not prepared for, and it quite unnerved me; I asked, therefore, for reflection. My consent was given, but with regret, for I felt that the much-loved occupation of my life would practically be ended."

Simonds's lifetime at the school was rewarded by warm thanks and a good pension, and the RCVS recognised professional stature by electing him one of its first British Honorary Associates. He was the single surviving signatory to the 1844 Charter.

A less tranquil twilight faced Thomas Walton Mayer, the only other man living who had been intimately associated with the first Charter. It will be recalled that the Mayers, father and son, had been the powerhouse of the Charter movement, the latter a dynamic secretary of the organising committee. In May 1840 *The Veterinarian* had written that "our children's children will have to thank them."

In August 1883 the son, now sixty-eight, addressed a heart-breaking letter to "The President, Vice-Presidents, Council, and Members of the Royal College of Veterinary Surgeons. Gentlemen, — It is with feelings of the deepest regret and greatest reluctance that I find myself compelled to place my present position before my professional brethren, and to appeal to their sympathy and support . . . the necessity has not arisen through want of prudence on my part . . . The Editors of *The Veterinarian* have kindly consented to receive donations."

It was an appeal for charity.

The response, some £70, was palliative only, and the unhappy man wrote a few months later to the RCVS asking if a donation he had made many years previously to initiate a College Building Fund could be returned to him. Discussion of this request at a meeting of the RCVS Council on 2nd October 1884, makes bitter reading.

"The application . . . by Mr T.W. Mayer . . . was next considered.

Mr Taylor said . . . the Council had no power to accede to the request, and moved that the money be not refunded.

Mr Cartwright seconded the motion.

Professor Robertson said that Mr Mayer had occupied a very important position in the profession prior to the Charter of 1844 being obtained. He had exerted himself to a considerable extent to get that Charter, and had expended his own money . . . all he asked . . . was to refund the amount out of a surplus which remained over from the money required to procure the Charter . . .

Mr Taylor asked if he did not derive an income from the Government.

Professor Robertson said . . . some nine shillings a day . . .

Mr Wragg said that . . . Mr Mayer was afraid of being made a bankrupt, and bankruptcy would mean a stoppage of his pension, and £40 or £50 would put him right again.

Professor Pritchard considered that the Council had no power to refund the money.

Mr Greaves suggested that, out of respect . . . a committee should be formed to receive individual subscriptions . . .

The Chairman remarked that, however worthy of consideration the suggestion might be, it was one outside the official duties of the Council, but might be acted upon by any individual member."

Thomas Walton Mayer, without whom there would have been no Charter in 1844, was abandoned by the children's children.

He died in 1887.

*   *   *

The 1876 Charter gave the RCVS power to appoint a Secretary outside the profession, and when Secretary Henry Coates, veterinary surgeon, resigned for health reasons in 1880, he was replaced by non-veterinary Arthur William Hill. Coates had served the RCVS well for eighteen years.

The versatility required of a Secretary of the RCVS, and the unpredictability of his responsibilities, are underlined by Secretary Hill's receipt two years later of unsolicited packets of pig powders. He explained to the Council that these had been delivered to the RCVS because although insufficiently addressed, they carried labels bearing the College Crest and the words 'Royal College of Veterinary Surgeons, London.' The Post Office had accepted the RCVS as consignor. The packets had been sent "to persons all over the country by a member of the Royal College." Secretary Hill sought Council's guidance, as he personally had no pressing need for pig powders.

In discussion, it was noted that "it was a very common thing for the veterinary surgeons of Great Britain to issue their letters with stamps similar to that on the letter in question," and Secretary Hill explained that he had frequently told Members "they would have to pay a guinea a year" (to the Inland Revenue) for the privilege of using the College Crest on professional stationery. President Fleming "thought the practice pursued by the gentleman in question was most reprehensible," but Councillor Cartledge claimed him as "a personal friend . . . and a respectable member of the profession." He undertook to have a private word with him. Clearly, in 1882 not everyone found unsolicited pig powders incompatible with professional dignity.

Of all Secretary Hill's problems — from the day of his appointment — the most urgent was to provide the RCVS with adequate accommodation in place of the second-class dwelling house in Red Lion Square, that in July 1883 was declared by the District Surveyor to be in so dangerous a state that "it was doubtful if Mr Hill could with safety remain with his family." Indeed, the 1882 and 1883 Annual General Meetings had been held in London hotels, because it was feared that the RCVS house might collapse under the press of the hundred or so people likely to attend.

The Hill family did not move out for another year, but by July 1884 even the stoical Secretary had to admit that the house "was really not fit for habitation. The domestic arrangements were imperfect" and "the place was deluged" whenever there was a shower of rain.

The tale of finding adequate covering for RCVS heads has elements of a saga.

The RCVS was nine years old before it acquired a permanent home. The early years in the unsavoury surroundings of the Freemasons' Tavern have been described, and satisfaction was considerable when No. 10 Red Lion Square was acquired in 1853. The lease had only twenty-one years to run, but that allowed ample time to find more suitable accommodation.

At the Annual General Meeting in 1868, however, fourteen years later, President Field was caught left-footed by Mr Boughton who wished to know "what had been done with the view" of "removal of the College to a more suitable locality." The President "said he was afraid he could not give much information on the point," and added that "the College funds were so small that they could ill afford to launch out in that direction." Mr Boughton considered "the present situation of the College was not one that was at all becoming to the profession," but his offer towards a Building Fund of "£5 a year for the remaining seven years of the lease," was soon forgotten.

After four more inactive years, with the end of the lease in sight, Councillor Fleming believed "that if a suitable appeal were made to the profession, sufficient funds would be obtained to enable the College to move into a respectable residence." A Building Fund was established a few months later, based on the original donation in 1849 by Thomas Walton Mayer of £37.14.7d, worth now, with interest, £64.17.1d. Contributions were personally solicited from every member of the profession, but only some £1300 had been collected by 1875, mostly in sizeable amounts from a small number of people. Fortunately the landlord agreed to a three-year lengthening of the lease, with further extension if necessary, but the likelihood seemed remote that private subscriptions would produce the money required for even modest improvement over existing accommodation.

It was agreed, therefore, after some heart-searching, to seek help from the Government. On 4th October 1876 a committee was appointed to "draw up a memorial to the Government, in regard to assistance in providing a suitable house and building for a museum." The fact that gestation of this memorial occupied twenty months indicates the reluctance with which the RCVS sought help outside the profession. The final document, written by Fleming, extolled the contribution of the profession to the welfare of the Nation, and emphasised that the RCVS had unimpeachable motives in presenting this "appeal, for the first time, to Her Majesty's Government for countenance and support in its laudable desire to still further benefit the country by continuing to improve veterinary education." The request was for "either a building which would meet the requirements of the Royal College, to be maintained at the cost of the corporation, or a sum of money to provide such premises."

It is difficult to believe that the RCVS really imagined that this overwritten document would persuade Treasury gentlemen to reach for the till. However, in 1878 President Fitzwygram led the RCVS deputation to an interview granted by the Duke of Richmond, Lord President of the Council. His Grace listened attentively, agreed the claim for help with housing was strong, coming as it did from so honourable a profession, and replied in bureaucratic jargon that was unequivocal in meaning: "In the present state of the Exchequer, and having regard to present demands which are being made by the present crisis on the National Funds, I fear I must say that the present is not a favourable opportunity of pressing your claims."

There must have been some unusually insensitive members of the RCVS Council at that time (Fleming, certainly), for hope of Government help was not immediately abandoned. A few months later the Council exposed itself to further rebuff by seeking "gratuitous use of one of the public buildings." But "there were none such available."

Towards the end of 1879, No. 16 Fitzroy Square cast a feeble ray across a lowering sky. A deputation pronounced it "far more eligible" than No. 10 Red Lion Square. To cover doubts about 'style' and 'frontage' expressed by a minority of Councillors, however, it was agreed to advertise for a property acceptable in all respects.

Advertisement produced nothing. A suitable property in Bedford Square was far beyond the cash available, and, in any case, "the inhabitants in the square would not like a public building in their midst." So, with minimal enthusiasm, negotiations were started for No. 16 Fitzroy Square, but almost immediately "the solicitor . . . expressed . . . doubts as to the genuineness of the title," and the deal was off.

It was now 1880, with the Red Lion Square lease extending on an *ad hoc* basis, the building becoming ever more dilapidated, and mould thriving in a dank museum. The next move, at a Council meeting in December, initiated by George Fleming (now President), who "with the assistance of a surveyor and architect" had "searched over London far and wide," was a proposal to raise within the profession £5000 in £5 shares, at three per cent interest, to buy a chapel in Tavistock Place, of which the "ground and building afforded ample space for a college such as they desired." A deputation to the site before launching the proposition took fright, however, over-ruled the President, and decided that "no steps should be taken to obtain a building until the finances of the College had so increased as to justify such a procedure." Thrift, no doubt, but achieving nothing. President Fleming did not enthuse.

With the Veterinary Surgeons' Act of 1881 occupying all hearts and minds, there was no alternative to suffering Red Lion Square in silence for another year. In 1882, however, the possibility of Government sponsorship for an RCVS building was resurrected by Fleming (re-elected President), whose success with the Act had boosted in-born self-esteem to an extent that made everything possible, the Fleming way. He would be backed by Earl Spencer, Lord Aberdare and others who had forged the Act. Certainly he succeeded in marshalling a galaxy of starlets to meet Earl Spencer, Lord President of the Privy Council Office, on 26th April

1882. There were over fifty noblemen and gentlemen "representative of agriculture, sanitary science, general science, public health, medicine, surgery, pathology, zoology, physiology, botany, chemistry, hippology and humanity."

Fleming spoke to a memorial previously presented.

Earl Spencer said: "I have carefully studied it."

Others urged Government grace for this worthy cause.

Earl Spencer said: "I will lay your petition and . . . interesting remarks . . . before my colleagues."

The RCVS received a Treasury reply dated 16th May 1882:-

"Sir,

I have laid before the Lords Commissioners of Her Majesty's Treasury your letter of 6th instant (72,397), forwarding a memorial addressed to the Lord President of the Council by the Royal College of Veterinary Surgeons, praying that the Government will be pleased to make a grant to the Council of the College to assist them in obtaining an edifice more suitable to the purposes of the institution than that which they at present occupy. I am to request that you will state to the Lord President that the memorial, etc., has been carefully considered, but my Lords regret that they cannot accede to the application for a grant to the Royal College of Veterinary Surgeons.

My Lords are deeply conscious of the importance of the study of diseases of animals as bearing on human diseases, and they are confident the zeal of the veterinary surgeons of the country will not allow this study to languish because it does not receive the doubtful benefit of public assistance.

The precedents to which attention is called in the memorial belong to another generation, and, as is confessed, have not recently been followed.

Sgd. Leonard Courtney"

Sympathy for President Fleming and his Council? Slight only, for any bookmaker would have offered five hundred to one against.

It took disintegration of the house and capitulation by Secretary Hill to reveal the obvious, expressed by Thomas Greaves (not the fastest of thinkers) at a Council meeting on 29th July 1884: "To have a new building erected on the present site."

The freehold was purchased without difficulty, architect's plans were approved, tenders sought, and work started within months. Indeed, progress was so rapid that a Foundation Stone ceremony planned to coincide with the 1885 Annual General Meeting was cancelled to avoid checking the momentum. The formal opening was on 6th April 1886, marked by President Roalfe Cox's luncheon for his Councillors "in the museum room." A few weeks later *The Veterinary Journal* proudly reported the: "Forty-third Annual General Meeting held on Monday, May 3rd 1886, at the New Building of the Royal College, Red Lion Square, W.C."

*   *   *

A historically important British National Veterinary Congress was held in "the beautiful and commodious rooms of the Society of Arts" in London on 20th and 21st July 1881. The congress had been proposed in a letter of November 1880 to *The Veterinary Journal*, signed by seven veterinarians led by George A. Banham. Attention was drawn to the forthcoming International Medical Congress in London, in which, it was emphasised, the veterinary profession *must* be interested, "especially in such matters as meat and milk inspection, and the relations of diseases of man to those of other animals." The proposed veterinary congress would discuss a range of scientific and professional matters, and the authors of the letter hoped that *The Veterinary Journal* would find space for "any correspondence on this subject." Editor Fleming was pleased to encourage so worthy a venture, and, in due course, was equally pleased to be President of the congress.

The objective was achieved of bringing together a large number of veterinary surgeons "not only from England, Ireland and Scotland, as well as the Army, but also from our Colonies," and providing a forum for discussion. The historic moment came when the talk was almost over. George Banham had circulated a pamphlet entitled, "Suggestions for the Formation of a British National Veterinary Association;" this became a resolution: "A British National Veterinary Association would be advantageous to the veterinary profession. A committee shall be formed to consider the subject and frame rules for its guidance."

In this manner was born the National Veterinary Association, that grew into the National Veterinary Medical Association, eventually to be named the British Veterinary Association.

*   *   *

An indication has been given of the revolution that followed the bacteriological discoveries of Pasteur and Koch. In the 1880's many other people were thinking, watching, experimenting in other fields. Army veterinary surgeon Griffith Evans described in *The Veterinary Journal* of

1881 the first-ever lethal trypanosome, a blood parasite, the cause of surra of horses in India. It is irrelevant now that Evans was treated with scorn by his seniors, for he is remembered for ever in the name of the parasite *Trypanosoma evansi*. In 1884 *The Veterinary Journal* gave a short history of artificial insemination, commenting: "We are not aware that it has been attempted to any extent in animals, though there is no reason why it should not at least be partially successful." In the same year the same journal carried an article on rickets, linking the disease with defective diet. Again, there was the novel treatment after loss of blood of intravenous infusion of salt solution, forerunner of the life-saving saline-drip. In 1885 several authors described cocaine as a local anaesthetic, marvelled at painless operations on conscious animals, and only regretted the "extremely high price . . . two shillings per grain."

The daily round in veterinary practice continued to be dominated by lame or colicky horses, by cows that could not calve, by pigs that would not eat, but discoveries breathed new interest, lifted cases above routine. Let's try that new idea! What was it Pasteur said?

Soon the Dear Queen would reach her Golden Jubilee. The first veterinary Charter had been "in the seventh year of our reign." Not a few remembered it.

In retrospect, another world. Another world in the future, too?

CHAPTER 11

Three new veterinary journals

New worlds, new ideas, new people.

In 1881 Fitzwygram and Fleming had given the profession its Act of deliverance from thraldom. Their part was nobly played. Thereafter, Fitzwygram backed away from the veterinary scene, in 1885 became Conservative Member of Parliament for Fareham in Hampshire, and, although still interested in veterinary matters, was not again involved in the profession's politics. Fleming, by contrast, could not yield to others. In 1886, unwisely and in an atmosphere of acrimony, he allowed himself to be elected for a fifth term as President of the RCVS. This compulsion to be big, big, big spoiled the earlier image of the selfless toiler. A possible explanation for increasing megalomania is that in 1884 he suffered several months of "mental breakdown," the consequence of multitudinous literary undertakings. Arrogance and ill-humour saddened his contemporaries, and infuriated younger men whom he tried to dominate.

Two of the younger men were William Hunting and John McFadyean.

Hunting was born in London in 1846, son of a groom about to enter the London veterinary school. On gaining his diploma, father Charles Hunting settled his family in South Hetton, County Durham, where he became a go-ahead practitioner and an authority on pit ponies. Part of William's schooling was at Edinburgh Academy; then, when seventeen, he became a student at John Gamgee's New veterinary school in that city. Gamgee and Charles Hunting were friends, William an enthusiastic pupil, under the Gamgee spell, soaking up not only technical knowledge, but also the philosophy and imagination of that brilliant brain. In due course, Hunting became an exceptional clinician and an expert on glanders in horses; the first article in Fleming's new *Veterinary Journal* of 1875 was by Hunting on that disease. He had a flair for simple, logical expression, spoken or written, and a sense of fun that pricked many a pompous bubble. He was a warm and generous man, and as stout a supporter of truth as opponent of chicanery. By the 1880's, in practice in London, he was well known throughout the profession. In 1888 he founded *The Veterinary Record*.

John McFadyean, seven years younger than Hunting, was born at Barrachan near Wigtown in Galloway, where his father was a tenant farmer of modest means. He attended the village school, then for two years the recently opened Ewart Institute in Newton Stewart, a first-class seminary in the Scottish three-R's tradition. At sixteen he left school and worked for five years as a paid hand on his father's farm. In 1874, aged twenty-one, there was enough money for him to attend the Edinburgh veterinary school, from which he obtained his diploma (plus medals and prizes) two years later. Principal Walley offered, and McFadyean accepted, a post to teach anatomy in the school, but, enthralled by the researches of Pasteur and Koch, he determined to continue his studies in Edinburgh university. In 1877 he enrolled for courses in medicine and science, to run concurrently. Of the bread and butter provided by the lectureship in anatomy, the bread was used to maintain bodily function, and the butter to pay class fees.

After five years of incredible toil, McFadyean graduated in medicine in 1882 and in science a year later. This period of study covered the great discoveries announced by Koch and Pasteur at the 1881 International Medical Congress in London. McFadyean was the first specifically trained British veterinary pathologist, for the courses in medicine and science were but means to the end of acquiring instruction in pathology and bacteriology. He never practised medicine, and was first and always a veterinary surgeon. By the mid-1880's, through his students, through papers presented to societies, but especially through his textbook, "The Anatomy of the Horse: A Dissection Guide," he too was well known in the profession. Like Hunting, McFadyean wrote and spoke succinctly. He treasured his laboratory, and his skill as a microscopist was supreme. Truth to McFadyean was absolute. Unlike the gregarious Hunting, McFadyean enjoyed friends in smaller numbers. He was unsmiling in demeanour, scathing in condemnation, apparently aloof, but eyes that missed nothing — not one thing — could twinkle too. In 1888 he launched a new periodical, *The Journal of Comparative Pathology and Therapeutics*.

It is happy and remarkable that the story of the veterinary profession (initially insignificant in numbers and still small), should have been chronicled, year in and out, from conception, through gestation, infancy and childhood to whatever stage the present may be styled. It is happier and more remarkable that the chroniclers should have been not only

veterinary surgeons, but also scribes with a persistent urge to communicate. Had they not been veterinary surgeons, authenticity might have
been in doubt, but the tale has been told through the eyes of those who
were there. *The Veterinarian* monthly from 1828; *The Veterinary
Journal* monthly from 1875; now *The Veterinary Record* weekly, and
The Journal of Comparative Pathology and Therapeutics quarterly,
from 1888.

Hunting's *Veterinary Record* was not a sudden decision. Indeed, for a
long time he had been considering a weekly journal based on recording
the proceedings of meetings of the various veterinary medical associations. In 1881 he put to the associations the suggestion that "sufficient
literary matter would be forthcoming to keep a weekly record going," but
the reception was lukewarm. Five years later, William Mulvey addressed
the North of England association on the need for "a new veterinary
journal . . . that would more thoroughly represent the views and opinions
of the veterinary medical associations, and, in addition contain articles
on comparative pathology and scientific research." Again, however, the
matter dropped, and was not revived until 1887 when the National Veterinary Association at last seemed positive in the resolution: "That the
time has arrived for the profession to be represented by a Weekly Scientific Journal, published under the auspices of the National Veterinary
Association — representing the Veterinary Medical Associations of
Great Britain — and supported by a registered staff of contributors."

Intentions were good, but the will was weak.

As nothing had happened by mid-1888, Hunting took a deep breath,
borrowed a little money (it is alleged), and started *The Veterinary
Record* as a private enterprise. It was an immediate success. Twelve pithy
pages of news and comment, well printed and well written. Just what the
practitioners ordered. There was to be particular emphasis on clinical
material. Hunting urged his colleagues to record their cases: "Careful
observation makes a skilful practitioner, but his skill dies with him."

McFadyean's *Journal* was entirely different from Hunting's *Record*.
There had been speculation among colleagues as to the likely format of
this new journal, for by this time McFadyean was involved in the politics
as well as the education and the science of the profession. He took all by
surprise by launching the journal, without preface, warning, or explanation, with a highly technical paper written by himself: "The Pathology of
Haemoglobinuria (Azoturia) of Horses." Its scientific worth was obvious,
but reader-appeal was in doubt because of the technicalities involved.
Woven into the paper, however, were comments that everyone understood: "One nowhere finds a writer who has the courage to say 'The

pathology of this affection is quite unknown; let us be slow to theorise regarding it until we have ascertained more than is known regarding its morbid anatomy.' " Or: "The custom of giving forth as ascertained and demonstrated facts what are merely speculative theories, has done immeasurable harm in retarding investigation."

No reader of that first paper doubted the determination of its author to make scientific investigation part of the veterinary way of life.

In addition to the solid science of original articles, and reprints and abstracts from many sources, especially France and Germany, each number of McFadyean's *Journal* contained three or four editorials, in which every aspect of the investigation and control of animal diseases was critically examined. McFadyean had an extra sense that could detect the importance, or futility, of an investigation in its earliest stages. In this manner readers were kept up-to-the-minute with discoveries of veterinary moment. In those early years of scientific investigation of animal diseases, every important advance was recognised by McFadyean and passed to his readers. He could be crushing in criticism, but was always fair, stating each side of a case before wielding the axe. An early editorial, for example, dealt with the suggestion by a medical officer of health to the Local Government Board that human diphtheria might be due to infection from pigeons, fowls, turkeys, pheasants, cats, pigs, sheep or horses. Cases of diphtheria had been noted in people who had handled sick animals. McFadyean wrote: "These observations of Dr Turner will materially lighten the labours of medical practitioners in tracing the infections in cases of diphtheria. Let them merely enquire whether the patient (or one of his relatives) has been near a horse or other lower animal. When he gets an affirmative reply, he need not further pursue his investigations . . . but we have already quoted enough of this absurd paper." It was no wonder that McFadyean's editorials became compulsive reading throughout the land.

Hunting and McFadyean, then, in their individual styles, caught the mood of the profession as it moved into the last decade of the nineteenth century. Both publications welcomed new ideas . . . and excellence.

*   *   *

Before leaving the 1880's, tribute must be paid to a little-known veterinary surgeon whose name is a household word. John Boyd Dunlop, of farming stock, Scot of Scots, with Boyds, Roxburghs and Stewarts in his pedigree, was born at Dreghorn in Ayrshire in 1840. At school he showed aptitude for mathematics, but elected to be a veterinary surgeon. He gained his diploma from Dick's school in 1859, and became a successful practitioner in Belfast. He had inventive talent, and was especially interested in the mechanics of movement. In 1887 he discovered that a wooden wheel with an air-filled rubber-and-canvas tube secured to the rim, ran faster and more easily across the stable-yard than a similar wheel with a solid rim. He made and fitted what he called "air-tyred" wheels to his son's tricycle, and found that they were much more efficient than wheels with solid tyres. These were the preliminary steps to fitting "air-tyred" wheels to a bicycle in 1888. This invention, a vital ingredient of the development of the motor-car, was described years later by Sir George Beharrell, Chairman of the Dunlop Rubber company, as "the greatest contribution to transport since the invention of the wheel itself."

Dunlop became a millionaire? Indeed no. He continued to practise as a veterinary surgeon, and in 1891 was specially commended by the Belfast Street Tramways Company "for his skill . . . in successfully combating a serious outbreak of 'pink-eye' among the horses, 561 out of 788 being affected and only eight died." 'Pink-eye' (equine viral arteritis) is an infectious disease of horses, controlled by isolation and careful nursing. Dunlop resigned from the Board of the Pneumatic Company in 1895. His last thirty years were spent in Dublin, and at his death quotation was made from Pope's epitaph to Addison:-

"Who broke no promise, serv'd no private end,
   Who gain'd no title, and who lost no friend."

*   *   *

In 1890 Robert Koch — that incredible man — made even larger headlines than in 1876 (anthrax), 1881 (pure cultures of micro-organisms), and 1882 (identification of the tubercle bacillus). For some time he had been working in strict secrecy, and it was rumoured that there had been an important discovery. The Tenth International Medical Congress was to be in Berlin that summer, and a number of Very Important People indicated to Koch that a major announcement would be appropriate, not only for science but also for Germany. He was put under tremendous pressure to reveal the results of his secret experiments. In vain he pleaded that they were incomplete, that he needed more time, that he preferred to make no statement at all. That, he was told, was out of the question, because he was to be the focal point of the Congress.

Rumour of a great revelation brought scientists to Berlin in their multitudes. Some thousands assembled in the Renzi circus amphitheatre for Koch's address. He told them that for sometime he had been seeking a cure for tuberculosis. At long last, after many failures, he had found a substance that prevented growth of tubercle bacilli not only in test-tubes, but also in the animal body.

Pandemonium!

Koch's appeal for caution in interpretation of these preliminary results in guinea-pigs, was lost in a frenzy of applause.

Then came letters, in thousands, appeals from individuals, petitions from Governments begging for the magic substance, or its recipe, so that sufferers could be saved. Overwhelmed, Koch was forced to close his laboratory to all visitors.

A special meeting of the RCVS Council on 25th November 1890 is explicable only against this phrenetic background. It was called to consider two motions in the name of Councillor (ex-President) Sir Henry Simpson. In summary (because, like Councillor Thomas Greaves, Sir Henry avoided simple sentences), he moved that the RCVS should vote a first instalment of £250 for investigation of "Dr Koch's recent discovery for the cure of Tuberculosis," and should dispatch to Berlin "a gentleman of acknowledged eminence in the Veterinary Profession" who would "place himself in communication with Dr Koch," and thus ensure early and authentic information for the RCVS. It was time, said Sir Henry, to "make an investigation . . . entirely on our own account." What precisely the RCVS was to do was not defined, nor was it mentioned that there was no commitment in the Charter to 'scientific investigation.'

Sir Henry Simpson had not recovered from the shock of being knighted at the time of Queen Victoria's Golden Jubilee, when, by chance, he was Mayor of Windsor (in addition to professional attendance on Her Majesty's buck-hounds), and had organised the Jubilee celebrations involving Windsor Castle. That made him the second British veterinary surgeon to receive the accolade. The first, Charles McMahon who had emigrated to Australia, was knighted for services as Speaker in the House of Assembly in the State of Victoria.

Sir Henry now lived on a higher plane than his fellow RCVS Councillors, so that he could properly say of Koch: "When we remember that he has not only been taken in hand by men of his own profession, but that the Emperor of Germany, who is very far-seeing for a young man, has absolutely had him in his presence and conferred the highest distinction on him . . . I think that ought to go very largely to reassure us that Dr Koch is . . . on that right track." Sir Henry then revealed that he personally could arrange access to Dr Koch's barricaded laboratory: "I ventured the other day to write to Prince Christian, at Berlin . . . I have known him for twenty years . . . he received my letter which he read to the Empress Frederick . . . she would show my letter to Dr Koch and

James Beart Simonds

1810–1904

Signatory to the 1844 charter. Principal of the London veterinary school. Founder in 1865 of the Government veterinary department

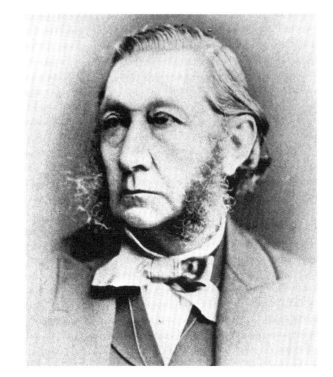

RCVS

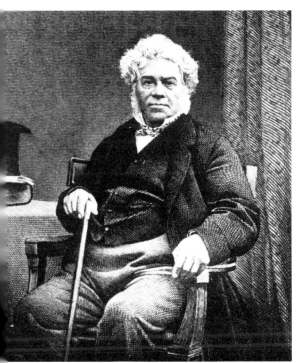

William Dick

1793–1866

Signatory to the 1844 charter. Founder in 1823 of the Edinburgh veterinary school

RCVS

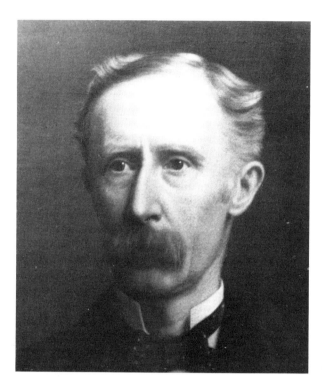

Sir Frederick Fitzwygram

1823–1904

In 1879 negotiated abolition of the Highland certificate

George Fleming

1833–1901

Architect of the 1881 Veterinary Surgeons Act

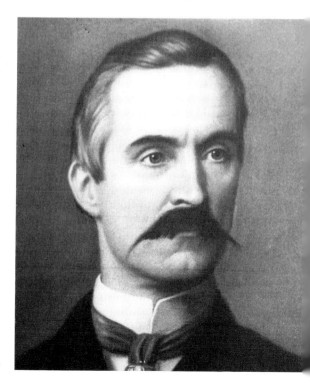

Sir John McFadyean

1853–1941

Principal of the London veterinary school and founder of British veterinary research

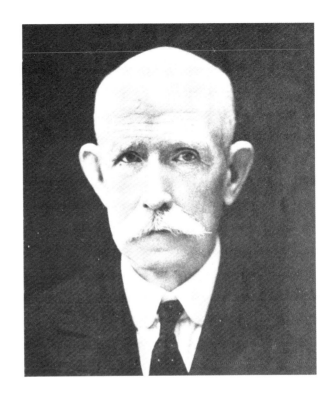

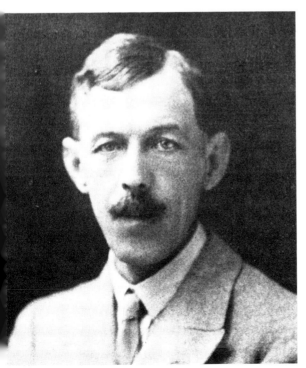

Sir Stewart Stockman

1869–1926

McFadycan's son-in-law. Chief Veterinary Officer. In 1917 established the Government central veterinary laboratory

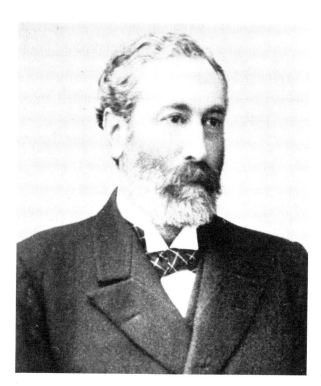

William Hunting

1846–1913

In 1888 founded *The Veterinary Record*

RCVS

Aleen Cust

1875–1937

In 1922 became first lady member of The Royal College of Veterinary Surgeons

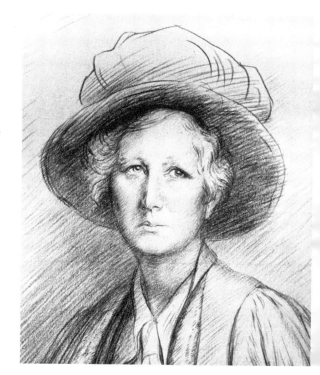

RCVS

endeavour to make an early arrangement . . ."

Having indicated the circles in which he now moved, Sir Henry hoped his motions would be carried unanimously. However, three years of knighthood had blurred his recollection of the veterinary virtue of rustic commonsense. Councillor Cox thought the proposition premature. Councillor Hunting said that all the fuss was due to "Royal Heads, who know nothing whatever of pathology, Crown Princes and newspaper reporters." Hunting objected to "our collectively calling our personal curiosity 'scientific investigation.' " Councillor Penberthy said that "Dr Koch will, under no circumstances, to anyone whatever, divulge the secret."

Sir Henry stepped sideways. Very well, let them not send anyone to Berlin immediately, but form a small committee with power to spend £250 should there be some sudden, unforeseen development. Agreed.

There was indeed unforeseen development. The December 1890 number of McFadyean's *Journal* contained a summary of an attempt by Koch to rationalise the distortions by others of his alleged cure for tuberculosis. He could not yet describe the material with which he was working, but would do so immediately his experiments were completed. In the meantime, he could say that healthy people did not respond to injection of the material, but its injection into tuberculous people caused a marked local and general reaction. He commented: "I think I am justified in saying that the remedy will . . . form an indispensible aid to diagnosis."

Events moved with break-neck speed. Shortly afterwards, Koch described his 'fluid.' It was simply a concentrated liquid culture of the tubercle bacillus, filtered to remove bacterial cells, so easy to make that it could immediately be tested all over the world; at first it was called 'tuberculinum,' but soon 'tuberculin.' Surely no substance has been more extensively examined in so short a time. Within months it became clear that tuberculin was not a cure for tuberculosis, but Koch's claim that it could be an aid to diagnosis was upheld. Tuberculin was first injected into cattle at the Russian Dorpat Institute in December 1890. There was no reaction in two normal animals, but three with tuberculosis showed a marked rise in temperature. The first test of tuberculin in Britain was by McFadyean in Edinburgh, the results being given in: "Experiments with Tuberculinum on Cattle," published in the March 1891 number of his *Journal*. Thus began the veterinary crusade against bovine tuberculosis.

The 'scientific investigation' proposed for the RCVS by Sir Henry Simpson, was overtaken by events. The committee met, however, on 18th February 1891, and voted £25 to each school for experiments with tuberculin. Sir Henry lost interest when his personal contact with the German

Royal Family was no longer relevant. He had to deal with more pressing matters.

Particularly in Sir Henry's mind was the RCVS meeting of 7th April 1891. A complaint against him as an examiner at the London school the previous December, had been lodged with the school's General Purposes Committee. It had reached the RCVS by a devious route, and was now discussed. In the practical examination, it was alleged, too many candidates were seen in one day, and "the examinations were in some cases conducted by candlelight."

Sir Henry had been forewarned of this criticism, to the extent of having prepared some thousands of words of outraged defence, and having submitted his resignation as an examiner. He recalled some points in detail, but of the candlelight accusation he said: "It is not a matter of absolute certainty to me whether I did not, with a view of giving a pupil a chance, towards the latter part of the afternoon bring a candle for the purpose of looking for a thrush or a corn." The true reason for his mortification was revealed in the comment: "I very much regret that such misleading remarks should have been addressed to a body of noblemen and gentlemen" (i.e. the Governors of the London school).

Some older members of the Council urged reconsideration of so grave a step as resignation, but Hunting said: "He tells you that he sent in this letter of resignation because we insulted him. I hope to goodness, that you will accept the resignation as his best reward."

Sir Henry refuelled his ego by declaring: "I cannot alter my decision."

The significance of this episode is in explanation of Sir Henry Simpson's opposition to a new RCVS Charter, essential for the advance of the profession.

The necessity for a new Charter arose out of the ninth clause of the Charter of 1876, which stated that ten years hence (1886) only Fellows of the RCVS could be elected to the Council. The idea had originated with Fitzwygram and Fleming as an incentive to higher education. The anticipated rush for the Fellowship diploma did not materialise, however, and with the decade to 1886 coming to an end, it was suddenly realised that election to Council would soon be restricted to a few individuals, and those not the ablest available.

The first call to action was at a meeting of the Royal Counties Veterinary Medical Association in Aylesbury on 28th November 1884, when a resolution was adopted to the effect that the ninth clause of the 1876 Charter should be rescinded. The point was picked up and approved by a number of other regional associations, but was resisted editorially by Fleming in *The Veterinary Journal* of May 1885. In July of that year, the

RCVS set up a committee under the chairmanship of Henry Simpson (not yet knighted) to examine the matter. At that time Simpson was in favour of action to remedy "what he thought an injustice to those members of the College who were not also Fellows."

The RCVS sought the opinion of Counsel C.E.H. Chadwyck Healey. He declared that after 23rd August 1886, by clause nine of the 1876 Charter, only Fellows, or members of the Council at the time of the 1876 Charter, could be RCVS Councillors, and that the clause could be rescinded only by another Charter or Act of Parliament.

Grumbling continued throughout the profession. The matter was brought to life by Hunting in *The Veterinary Record*. In September 1890 he urged the case for a new Charter, not only to rescind clause nine of the 1876 Charter, but also to prevent Councillors acting as examiners, and to have Vice-Presidents chosen from among elected Councillors, instead of, as hitherto, by addition to elected members. Thus, the examiners would no longer be judges of their own behaviour (a third of the Councillors were examiners), and Vice-Presidents would no longer be the particular friends of elected Councillors.

From the violent reaction of some seniors to these three proposals, each essential to impartial and top-quality government, it might have been supposed that the proposition was execution for a peccadillo. However, William Mulvey, practitioner in London, contemporary and friend of Hunting, proved this to be only the noise of an entrenched few. In November 1890, at his own expense, he circularised every member of the profession, asking if they were in favour of a new Charter to cover the proposals. The response, published in *The Veterinary Record* of 6th December 1890, was an overwhelming 'yes' for a new Charter — 978 in favour and 23 against.

Sir Henry Simpson's opposition to the new Charter was at first too subtle to be obvious. At the time of his resignation as an examiner in April 1891, however, he marked William Hunting (who had urged acceptance of his resignation) for high disfavour, and as Hunting was champion of the Charter it too could not be countenanced. By August 1891 he was talking of the profession casting aside "old and tried servants". In October, in discussion of a draft of the Charter, he was critical of the RCVS for "their not having studied the way in which municipal and other institutions in this country are conducted" and when, in December, at a meeting called specifically to affix the RCVS seal to the petition for the new Charter, his attempt to reopen discussion on its contents was resisted, he had "never received such treatment as today, except on one occasion

when I was insulted" (i.e. when his behaviour as an examiner was ques-
tioned).

The glove was off.

The fist was shown in March 1892 in an open letter sent for publicity to
The Veterinary Record, in which Sir Henry informed the profession that
he had "entered a protest against the Charter," now under consideration
by the Privy Council. However, he would be prepared to withdraw the
protest if "some reasonable concessions" were made "on matters of
detail." William Mulvey, to whom the letter was addressed, referred it to
the RCVS Council.

Hunting published a blistering editorial in *The Veterinary Record*:
"Sir Henry Simpson . . . stands forth to oppose the veterinary profession
single-handed . . . victorious or defeated, Charter or no Charter, he
stands to win — notoriety." Hunting was emphatic: "This is a critical era
in our corporate life."

That was not exaggeration. Sir Henry Simpson was a powerful man.
Knights were not for trifling with in the reign of Queen Victoria. Opposition to the Charter from a former President of the RCVS would be most
seriously considered by the Privy Council. It is to the utmost credit of
William Mulvey and William Hunting that they were unmoved by arrogance. To them, the profession was everything.

The climax was reached on 31st March 1892, at a meeting of the RCVS
Council convened specially to consider the "protest lodged by Sir Henry
Simpson against the grant of the Supplemental Charter."

Sir Henry had now passed the border of rationality. His protest was
that a new Charter would be "contrary to the true intent and meaning of
the Veterinary Surgeons' Act, 1881," would adversely affect "the status
and rights" of Existing Practitioners and Members and Fellows of the
RCVS, and so on, and so on, until President Lambert was asked: "Is there
any advantage in prolonging this discussion?" He replied: "I do not think
there is."

Sir Henry submitted two protests to the Privy Council. Their
Lordships sought clarification from the RCVS. This was provided after
long meetings on 7th and 20th April 1892. Sir Henry was permitted to
state his case *ad nauseam*, but it was now so bizarre as to be in places
unintelligible.

Then he resigned from the RCVS Council.

Sir Henry Simpson's protests to the Privy Council achieved nothing,
and the Charter was granted. His place in veterinary history is as a reflecting glass for a maturing RCVS. He was dealt with tactfully, fairly, firmly,
and with the consideration that his earlier contributions to the Council

required. Reasonable men bowed not to unreason, and were conscious of leadership of their profession.

On a happier note, an appointment of great consequence was made in 1892. In October of that year John McFadyean of Edinburgh became the first Professor of Pathology and Bacteriology at the London veterinary school.

CHAPTER 12

Unprofessional conduct

The appointment of John McFadyean to the London school in 1892 was not only as first Professor of Pathology and Bacteriology, but also as first Dean.

The new Chair was supported by an annual grant of £500 (dating from 1890) from the Royal Agricultural Society of England, emphasising yet again the important relationship between the Society and the school. It will be recalled that William Youatt had urged the Society, in its earliest days, to include support for veterinary science in its terms of reference. This was agreed, and the undertaking had been faithfully honoured. It will be recalled, also, that in 1842 the Society had endowed at the London school a Chair in Cattle Pathology, to which James Beart Simonds was appointed. The Society's interest in, and financial support for, study of diseases of farm animals was vital in the development of veterinary science in Britain. In return, the school — Simonds in parti-cular — carried out many investigations for the Society, and from time to time presented to its members formal lectures on important diseases. Now, through the Society's munificence, John McFadyean brought to London unique expertise in the pathology of animal diseases. His train-ing in this new field far surpassed that of any other British veterinary surgeon, and the quality of his *Journal of Comparative Pathology and Therapeutics* (now four years old) reflected not only scientific ability, but also an understanding of veterinary science that could be matched only by a handful of men in other countries, Nocard in Paris, perhaps, Johne in Dresden, Bang in Copenhagen.

The new post of Dean had a more complex origin. It reflected the Governors' dissatisfaction with the school's performance, but also some uncertainty that McFadyean was the man to improve it. Principal Robertson had died suddenly in December 1887, and the Governors saw no obvious successor. Professor George Thomas Brown had excellent qualifications, but no wish to cease being Chief of the Veterinary Department of the Board of Agriculture. After consideration of the restricted field, however, Brown was appointed Principal on a part-time basis. It was an unsatisfactory arrangement, soon reflected in staff dissension and poor examination results.

A committee was appointed to investigate, and its highly critical report was considered at a meeting of the General Purposes Committee in November 1891. It was regretted "that the evidence . . . has clearly shown that the harmony and cordial co-operation necessary to secure the full efficiency of the teaching staff has not existed among the professors of the College." Governor Edgar March Crookshank, Professor of Bacteriology at King's College, London, then proposed "that a resident Dean should be appointed, responsible to the Principal and through him to the Council for the working of the school." It seemed a good idea, especially when someone wondered if McFadyean of Edinburgh might be interested. His reputation as scientist and teacher was established, and the only doubt was whether at thirty-eight he had the maturity to reorganise and control a complex community.

Principal Brown was instructed to ascertain on what terms — if any — McFadyean would come to London. The reply was £800 annually plus residence in the school. The Governors offered £600. By return of post, McFadyean repeated £800, or no move to London. The Governors agreed, impressed by the briskness of this young man.

Their selection of McFadyean was quickly justified. In weeks, order emerged out of confusion. Principal Brown was delighted to have the reins in competent hands, so that he could give full attention to his Government work. After some sixteen probationary months, Brown informed the Governors: "I am perfectly satisfied that it would be to the interests of the College that Professor McFadyean should act with an undivided responsibility."

As well as continuing to be Professor of Pathology and Bacteriology, and Dean, John McFadyean became Principal of the London veterinary school in February 1894.

McFadyean's translation from Edinburgh to London coincided with general realisation that reorganisation of veterinary education was urgently required. The veterinary world was in danger of drowning in the storm of exploding science. The course had been lengthened since the earliest days, examinations had become more searching and standards had been raised, but far too many inadequate men were still wriggling through. William Hunting was editorially scandalised in *The Veterinary Record* of 13th August 1892: "On another page will be found some examples of the certificates written by students" for the final examinations. "They are a disgrace to the profession."

He had a point.

One certificate declared: "I certify that I have this day exam. for . . . white Bony Mare 5 years old 4 white feet. Find that she has a splint off fore Curb, spavined near hind spavin off, and therefore in my opinion unsound."

Another: "This is to certify that I this day examined a dapelid Gray mare in the possession of . . . I find said animal aged also got both fore knees bumped & stiff & thereby unsound, also thickened fetlocks I also find fractured haunch on off side & thereby unsound & week spine over the lumber region I also find bone spavin on off hock & also unsound, & also calised Fetlocks & Thrush on both hind & Splint on off hind."

After due allowance for the technical obscurity of spavins, splints, curb, and thrush, the ignorance revealed by such certificates was professionally intolerable.

A consensus that review of veterinary education was essential, emerged from meetings of the Court of Examiners in December 1891. This stimulated the RCVS to assess the examination system, and to arrange in July 1892 a conference of teachers, examiners and members of the RCVS Council. There could be no more cogent proof of widening veterinary horizons. Such a conference would have been unthinkable a decade earlier, with schools and RCVS suspicious of each other's every move.

The conference was reported *in extenso* in *The Veterinary Record*; seventeen double-column pages of close type describing the existing veterinary curriculum, proposals for its improvement, and the comments of leading teachers. It is an illuminating document, catching the contemporary scene, reflecting the past, anticipating the future. The two most important conclusions were that the instruction now required by graduating veterinarians could not be compressed into less than four years, and that there must be written as well as oral examinations. It was agreed that each written examination would be of four questions in two hours. Test papers for the first written examinations were reprinted in *The Veterinary Record* for 20th May 1893, and the organisation was described as "a big job . . . carried out synchronously in Glasgow, Edinburgh and London . . . the result . . . a brilliant success." The first graduating examinations for a four-year course were in 1897, and the examiners noted "a marked improvement in the general proficiency of the candidates."

On McFadyean's departure from Edinburgh, two outstandingly able young men, both graduates of the Edinburgh school, took over his teaching responsibilities. Stewart Stockman became Professor of Pathology and Bacteriology, and Albert Mettam Professor of Anatomy. Principal Thomas Walley died in 1894. Walley had pulled the school together after Principal Williams's resignation in 1873 to set up the New Edinburgh school. Walley's major professional publication was in 1890, a "Practical Guide to Meat Inspection," one of the earliest books on the subject to be published in Britain. His successor was John Dewar, Professor of Surgery and Obstetrics at the school.

Concern in the 1890's for improvement in veterinary education, was matched by anxiety for the future of the Government's veterinary department, created to deal with the cattle plague catastrophe in 1865, with Simonds as Veterinary Adviser and Brown his Chief Inspector. At first it was called the Veterinary Department of the Privy Council Office; then, briefly, in 1866 the Cattle Plague Department, and later in the same year again the Veterinary Department. In 1883 it was submerged in the Agricultural Department of the Privy Council Office, but in 1889 surfaced as the Veterinary Department of the Board of Agriculture. When Simonds was appointed Principal of the London veterinary school in 1872, he was succeeded by Brown who gave outstanding service for twenty-one years, including highly efficient control of two more cattle plague invasions, in 1872 and 1877. When, aged sixty-five, he retired in 1893, his services were retained on a consultative basis (a rare occurrence in the Civil Service) for a further three years.

On Brown's official retirement in 1893, the veterinary world expected him to be succeeded by his competent first lieutenant Alexander Cope. Not so. No announcement of a successor was made.

There was no promotion for Cope, nor for William Duguid, the third veterinary surgeon in the Department. There were ominous whispers of "reorganisation." Then a new leader emerged, one Major Tennant, a retired soldier, who had been in administrative charge of travelling inspectors in Brown's Veterinary Department. That Department had now been replaced by an "Animals Division," of which Tennant was "Principal." In the words of *The Veterinary Record*, veterinary surgeons Cope and Duguid might now be "consulted when any of the directing officers recognised their inability to direct without the guidance of experts." The operative word in this comment was 'recognised,' for *The Veterinary Record* well knew that intellectual modesty is not a prerequisite for promotion in Government service. Major Tennant was unlikely to find his experience inadequate to control animal diseases. After all, had he not successfully deployed the travelling inspectors?

The RCVS, the whole profession was alarmed. Clearly, in spite of cattle-plague, swine-fever, foot-and-mouth disease, glanders, pleuro-pneumonia and rabies, the lesson had not been learned that veterinary surgeons are the people most likely to know about veterinary matters.

Early in April 1895 the RCVS sent a tough memorandum to the Board of Agriculture, setting out the facts and deploring the action taken. The reply, dated 19th April 1895, from T.H. Elliot, Secretary to the Board, "most cordially and fully" recognised "the great benefits which stock-owners and the public generally have derived from the researches and work of veterinarians" (i.e. under the system that had been abandoned), but considered that now "both private and official veterinarians will be in a position and be encouraged to extend their work and researches."

Wrestling with a pillow.

By good fortune, President of the Board of Agriculture Herbert Gardner, was replaced in mid-1895 by the Right Honourable Walter Long, M.P. The RCVS lost no time in again pressing their case, and sought a meeting with the new President of the Board to request that (a) The Veterinary Department be restored (b) The Department be under direction of a veterinary surgeon (c) The staff of veterinary officers be strengthened.

RCVS President J.F. Simpson met President Long on 6th February 1896. The Board of Agriculture's President was sympathetic, and promised to give the problem his attention.

After a remarkably brief pause (in bureaucratic terms), RCVS President Simpson announced in *The Veterinary Record* of 16th May 1896, with "the greatest pleasure and satisfaction," that "the President of the Board of Agriculture has consented to the restoration of the 'Veterinary Department' with a veterinary surgeon at its head as Chief Veterinary Officer."

An arrangement that has continued the same in essentials, if not precisely in name, ever since.

It is possible that in deciding to re-establish a Government Veterinary Department, Walter Long was influenced in favour of the veterinary profession by discussions on the Public Health (Scotland) Bill then before Parliament. Through the initiative of RCVS Solicitor Thatcher, and with the co-operation of many in the profession who sought help from Members of Parliament, an amendment had been introduced that gave veterinary surgeons "equal powers with medical officers or sanitary inspectors." Not only that, and of much greater importance, "in the definition clause of the Act the expressions 'veterinary surgeon' and 'qualified veterinary surgeon' were stated to mean a member of the Royal College of Veterinary Surgeons." This was a decision for which the RCVS had waited fifty-three years. It induced the President to write a letter of thanks to the Lord Advocate, and to be assured in reply: "I am gratified to find that your profession is satisfied." Thus, at last, Members of the RCVS were legally differentiated from those who refused to add MRCVS to their Highland certificate. It was not put into words, of course, but everyone knew that the handful of men who still walked with the ghost of William Dick could not now be qualified veterinary surgeons within the meaning of this Act.

*   *   *

It has been said that discussion among veterinary surgeons in general practice is synonymous with argument. Certainly, they are strong in personal opinions. The profession attracts — or perhaps makes — people who relish the challenge of off-beat problems. It was always thus, but never more so than for William Kirk, MRCVS, of London in January 1896. He was "visited by two French celebrities, who had just received a three-year-old bear direct from his country. The beast had never been handled," and the owners were "naturally very anxious to secure him in some way," in order to train him "for theatrical performances."

Setting aside the deplorable Victorian attitude to captive wild animals, the problem at that moment was how to handle a "bear fully grown, and of immense strength . . . enclosed in a cage 5 feet square, made of the stoutest timbers, and having an iron-barred door . . . The owner was able to feed the beast through these bars," but "any attempt . . . to secure him" caused him to "grasp the bars with his great paws and make the cage fairly shake."

Kirk was invited to put a collar on the animal, and a ring through its nose.

He recorded: "The whole business was fraught with difficulty." Besides, the men who asked him to risk limb, if not life, were foreigners. He requested a note absolving him from blame in case of mishap. M. Clement gave him *carte blanche*:-

> "January 15th, 1896
> I authorise Dr Kirk to act as he thinks proper in the matter of drugging and operating on grizzly bear, and hold him irresponsible for effect."

Kirk "pocketed the letter and left, intimating that I would return in half-an-hour. On the way to my surgery I purchased half-a-pound of honey in which . . . I mixed seven grains of morphia hydrochlorate."

Within the half-hour he faced the bear: "To my delight he licked up every spot. The effect was rapid . . . the most terrible . . . yells I ever heard . . . This stage of excitement passed . . . and he was then noticed to reel about and lost control of his forearms."

The cage was opened, a collar was put on the animal, and it was fully anaesthetised with a mixture of ether and chloroform "on my pocket handkerchief." The required ring was put into the snout, and "it was surprising . . . how quickly he recovered consciousness. He took no food that day, but an excellent breakfast next morning."

Kirk rounded off his report by considering the dose of morphia he had used: "I should imagine had I given three grains more there would have been no necessity for the anaesthetic." It cannot be supposed that this revised dose was ever tested, but no doubt in the future, in discussion with colleagues, William Kirk would have strong views on sedation of grizzly bears.

At precisely the time William Kirk was engaged with the bear, Frederick Hobday, dynamic young house-surgeon at the London veterinary school, was making history with a cat. His experience was reported in the March 1896 number of McFadyean's *Journal*, under the title: "The New Photography in Veterinary Practice." The article began: "The application of Roëntgen's rays to veterinary practice may seem somewhat in the future as regards the larger animals, but for the smaller ones it certainly is likely to prove of value." There was an excellent photograph showing a piece of metal embedded in a leg of the cat, taken by "Mr Sidney Rowland, B.A. . . . using a 3-inch spark given by a large induction coil and exciting one of the new 'X' ray vacuum tubes." The cat was "kept perfectly still by the aid of hobbles and chloroform," and the picture was obtained "after an exposure of two-and-a-half minutes." The piece of metal thus located was successfully removed.

This appears to be the earliest diagnostic X-ray picture in veterinary literature.

*   *   *

The sixth clause of the 1881 Veterinary Surgeons' Act dealt with dismissal from the Register of anyone found guilty of "conduct disgraceful to him in a professional respect." Nine years later a Hunting editorial in *The Veterinary Record* noted that "this clause has never yet been acted on," and suggested that it was time to try to define disgraceful professional behaviour. However, the difficulty — not to say delicacy — of the proposal was reflected in those nine inactive years, for, as in all professions, one man's crime is another's indiscretion.

Even before 1881 there had been an attempt to identify unprofessional activities, initiated at the RCVS Annual General Meeting of 1880 by Tom

Dollar, a tough Scotsman whose veterinary skill and parsimony had produced one of the great London practices. To general approval, he declared: "That the profession . . . consider that the time has arrived when the Council should embody in a series of resolutions what derelictions of conduct on the part of any of their members will subject them to the cognisance of the Council." It is a pity that a proposition so splendidly expressed proved untranslatable into practice.

The first real stimulus to consideration of action against professional misconduct was economic, not altruistic. Times were hard in both medical and veterinary practice in 1890, and competition acute. The medical press carried advertisements offering, in parts of London, medicine and advice for as little as two pence, and RCVS Councillor Cox declared at a meeting in April of that year that some veterinary surgeons were issuing circulars "in large numbers, first offering to do business at half the usual fees . . . reduced to one-third and even one-sixth of the recognised and established terms." He considered this conduct professionally disgraceful, and proposed (a) That the RCVS "take means to regulate the professional conduct of its Members" (b) That "for the guidance of the College" account should be taken of how the problem of professional behaviour was handled by The Royal Colleges of Physicians, and of Surgeons, and The Society of Apothecaries and The Pharmaceutical Society (c) That the RCVS should "acquire full power . . . to determine questions of proper professional conduct." With regard to the third item, he was immediately reassured that full powers already existed under the 1881 Act. Councillor Cox's views were strongly supported, but it was considered impossible to itemise unprofessional acts. Councillor Hunting warned, however, that "you only have an offence when you make a law."

"The motion was then put and carried."

Carried, certainly, but no action taken.

Almost exactly four years later, the RCVS Council again wondered how to deal with disgraceful professional conduct. This discussion was an echo of the earlier one, even to the extent that Councillors had to be reminded that by virtue of the 1881 Act *they* were to decide what constituted disgraceful conduct, and whether a name should be removed from the Register. Right of appeal was to the Privy Council. The stimulus for this discussion was the specific complaint that a Member was advertising his services and nostrums by blowing a hunting horn in the local marketplace. Councillor McFadyean voiced the opinion of all when he called this an example of "the more flagrant cases" of unprofessional advertising. It was agreed that action must be taken, and this time the statement of intent encouraged the Registration Committee to look closely at advertising, and to report several other unacceptable cases to the next Council meeting in April 1894. On the Solicitor's advice, it was agreed to warn the profession that advertising was now considered conduct disgraceful in a professional respect, and would be dealt with accordingly.

In 1896 'covering' joined advertising as professionally unacceptable. If a veterinary surgeon used an unregistered person to carry out duties that, to be properly executed, required veterinary knowledge and skill, he was said to be 'covering' that person. There was no resistance to this RCVS decision, once the profession was reassured that to employ unskilled labour in kennels or stables was not covering. This reform was overdue, for there were instances of registered and unregistered men in partnership as 'veterinary surgeons.'

By outlawing advertising and covering, the RCVS established beyond peradventure that membership of the profession involved not only privileges, but also responsibilities beyond the common law. Other restrictions, established gradually over the years, have been accepted as advances in professional integrity and service.

*   *   *

In 1897 there was as much rejoicing in veterinary as in more, or less, sophisticated circles, that Queen Victoria had reigned for sixty years. William Hunting reviewed the occasion in *The Veterinary Record* for 26th June: "Sixty Years Ago" recalled that "in 1837 every wretched animal that was submitted to veterinary treatment underwent a course of bleeding, physicing and blistering . . . there was no veterinary pathology . . . Professor Sewell asserted that bad feeding and ill usage might cause rabies in dogs . . . the most conscientious practitioner would never sew up the simplest . . . wound until he had filled it with some filthy greasy compound . . . everyone believed that a healthy sign was . . . when a wound 'mattered freely' . . . men with the mere ability to read and write with difficulty could enter the ranks . . . twelve months study was all that was demanded . . . the high position the veterinary profession has attained during the Victorian reign only marks its arrival at adolescence . . . State and public recognition come to those who are deserving."

George Thomas Brown, Consulting Veterinary Adviser to the Board of Agriculture, was, in Hunting's word, 'deserving,' and in January 1898 he became the first truly veterinary knight. The profession was delighted. This skilled microscopist, patient teacher, prescient adviser, and gifted administrator deserved well of his colleagues and his country. But Hunting, wise and generous, ended a congratulatory editorial: "Grateful as we are for the honour done to Sir George Brown, we cannot help saying that we should have been even more pleased if the veteran Professor Simonds had also been recipient of some mark of recognition."

The oversight was historical, however, not personal. At eighty-eight, James Beart Simonds belonged to a veterinary generation that would not presume to knightly dreams.

CHAPTER 13

Turn of the century — Universities and veterinary education

This brief review of British veterinary history has said little about veterinary surgeons in the Army, because their tale has been told by Major-General Sir Frederick Smith in: "A History of the Royal Army Veterinary Corps, 1796–1919." He has traced development of the earliest regimental system — in which individual veterinary surgeons were attached to individual regiments — into a unified service, named in 1881 the Army Veterinary Department. He has described the foundation in 1880 of the Army Veterinary School at Aldershot, where, in addition to education of veterinary personnel, studies were made on veterinary hygiene and physiology, and where, from 1888, lymph was prepared for vaccination against human smallpox. He has recalled official disinterest in the Department, that resulted in veterinary unpreparedness for the Boer War of 1899.

That horse-war on a vast scale is specially mentioned here, because of its impact on civilian veterinary surgeons in Britain. For the first time, there was a plea for veterinary help with a problem that was beyond Army resources.

The desperate Army position was revealed to the RCVS Council on 10th October 1901, by Colonel Duck, in command of the Army Veterinary Department: "We are in great need of first-class veterinary surgeons . . . we want them particularly for transport ships. We are sending . . . 10,000 a month horses to South Africa and we occasionally have severe losses. We want . . . good men . . . in charge of the horses. My object is to ask you gentlemen to . . . make it known throughout the profession . . . We give a bonus of £50 . . . and 3s. per head on every horse landed in South Africa, presuming the loss to be under $2\frac{1}{2}$ per cent; a bonus of 2s. for every horse landed, assuming the loss to be under 5 per cent; and a bonus of 1s., assuming the loss to be under 7 per cent . . . Assuming you

118

have a cargo of 1000 horses . . . a veterinary surgeon could get nearly £200 for a month's work."

This blood-curdling revelation shows that the non-veterinary Army Remount Department (*not*, be it emphasised, the Veterinary Department), accepted without severe disfavour a loss in transit of five per cent of horses shipped to South Africa. Thus, of Colonel Duck's estimated 120,000 embarked in a year, 6,000 might 'reasonably' be expected to die at sea.

Patriotism, and official indifference to disease and death of horses in the Boer War, stimulated some one hundred civilian veterinary surgeons in Britain to volunteer for service in South Africa. Among them was Stewart Stockman, who had succeeded McFadyean as Professor of Pathology and Bacteriology at the Edinburgh school. For him, and for others, the war in South Africa was a challenge beyond anticipation. They found not only sickly and wounded horses, but also, on every side, animal diseases of cause unknown. The experience gained by these men was of historical significance in developing the veterinary services needed to consolidate, and expand, the British Empire.

*   *   *

The story of veterinary education in Ireland was already a hundred years old when a school affiliated to the RCVS was opened in Dublin in 1900. It was not a continuous story, but is worthy of recall because the beginning is as clear as that of the Odiham Agricultural Society through which the London school was founded. On 1st August 1800 Royal assent was given to an Act of Parliament that provided the Royal Dublin Society with a considerable sum of money for, among other items, "buildings for a veterinary institution . . . paying a salary to a veterinary professor, and maintaining a veterinary institution." The Society had a clear conception of requirements for veterinary education: "Lectures . . . on the constitution, nourishment, diseases, cures and treatment of the horse . . . cattle, pigs, sheep, and dogs . . . a forge . . . ten boxes or loose stalls for invalid horses . . ." And so on, in great detail. Thomas Peall and George Watts were appointed professor and lecturer, and assistant professor and practitioner, respectively.

It is not clear for how long this veterinary education (far more liberal than that of the contemporary London school) continued, nor why it ended. An investigation by the Society sixty years later presumed that there must have been "a deficiency of funds." The same investigation, however, urged that "re-establishment of a veterinary department" attached to the Society "would prove of immense utility to the country."

The idea was developed on paper, but appears to have been financially impracticable.

Twenty years passed before the proposition was again mooted of a veterinary school for Ireland. On that occasion the RCVS was involved, because a licensing body was envisaged in addition to a teaching school. That was as unacceptable for Ireland as it had been for Scotland. The RCVS had never wavered in its belief that there must be only one licensing body for veterinary sugeons in Great Britain and Ireland. A Memorial dated 31st December 1880 submitted by the RCVS to His Excellency Earl Cowper, K.G., Lord Lieutenant of Ireland, urged that its diploma remain the "one portal system of admission to the Profession," and prayed "your Excellency to favourably entertain the urgent prayer of the Memorialists, that a Charter for a Licensing Veterinary College in Ireland be not granted." The Memorial had the support of a majority of the practising veterinary surgeons in Ireland, who agreed with the RCVS that although a teaching school would be welcome a licensing body would not.

In the event, it proved impossible to raise the money required to establish a school, and the matter was dropped. Not without regret, however, for there was a widespread wish for a veterinary school in Ireland.

In 1894 the first move was made to convert wish into reality. In April of that year the RCVS Solicitor informed the Council that: "In accordance with the instructions I received from the President, I have been watching . . . the application for a Charter for the foundation of a Veterinary College in Ireland . . . the scheme contemplates a teaching college only . . . the Chief Secretary for Ireland . . . has definitely promised . . . £15,000 towards formation of the College . . . they will affiliate themselves to the Royal College of Veterinary Surgeons."

As far as the RCVS was concerned, this was entirely satisfactory, but the Government grant of £15,000 caused umbrage north of the Scottish border. The Principals of the three Scottish schools — Walley, Williams and McCall — in an unusual display of absolute unanimity, informed the profession through a joint letter to *The Veterinary Record* that they considered it "a great injustice" to their schools "that they should now have to compete with an Irish Veterinary College, established and endowed with Government money." They had "no objection whatever to . . . a grant to an Irish veterinary college provided the veterinary colleges which have been successfully conducted all these many years be put on the same footing."

But there was nothing for the Scots.

Ireland now built her school in Dublin, for which a Charter was granted in 1895. Inauguration of the school was in 1900, and Albert Mettam, (who had been appointed Professor of Anatomy when McFadyean left the Edinburgh school) was the first Principal. The first examination was on 17th July 1901 in "one of the examination rooms" in the Royal University of Ireland, "for which no charge whatever was made." Mettam proved to be as able an administrator in Dublin as he had been teacher in Edinburgh, with the admirable attribute of saying little and doing much.

*   *   *

The adjective 'Victorian' began its journey towards the lexicon when the legendary Queen died in January 1901. Veterinary attitudes can still be 'Victorian' in the 'old-fashioned' sense, but the faintly derogatory connotation should be cautiously applied to veterinary matters. The greatest men in British veterinary history were Victorians. A handful of worthy leaders followed, but only in the footsteps of the masters. The independence and objectives of the profession were established by men born in Victorian days.

Three great veterinary surgeons died in the early years of King Edward's reign: George Fleming, Sir Frederick Fitzwygram, and James Beart Simonds.

George Fleming died in 1901, aged sixty-eight. He had retired from the veterinary scene (to Combe Martin in Devon) some years previously, except to remain an examiner for the RCVS. He had given up editorship of *The Veterinary Journal*, his literary work limited to revision of his numerous text-books. A sketch has been given of his early life, and his impact on the profession through the RCVS Council and the 1881 Veterinary Surgeons' Act has been recorded. It has been suggested that mental illness in 1884 contributed to the megalomania and irascibility of the last years of his life. It is distressing to recall the self-aggrandisement, the outbursts of ill-humour, the malicious libel actions, and the pointless rudeness that muddied his later years. Better to remember with gratitude the will-power that achieved the Veterinary Surgeons' Act, and the generosity that bequeathed to the RCVS some seven hundred volumes, many valuable and rare, collected in a lifetime by this talented, tormented man.

Frederick Fitzwygram and James Beart Simonds died in 1904, the former aged eighty-one and the latter ninety-four.

Fitzwygram's achievement of an armistice between the RCVS and the Highland and Agricultural Society has been described, the basis for the 1881 Veterinary Surgeons' Act. Mention has not been made, however, of the 'Fitzwygram Prizes' he established in 1875 to encourage veterinary education and colleagueship between the schools. Premiums totalling £100 were given annually to the three students, from any school, graduating with the highest number of marks, there being a minimum below which no prize was awarded. By a codicil to his will, dated 14th May 1903, Fitzwygram ensured that these prestigious prizes would be continued beyond his death. He was a good friend to the profession, particularly interested in education, as a Governor of the London school and through the Army's training establishment at Aldershot. As a baronet and wealthy land-owner, he might have been excused condescension towards contemporaries in a humble profession, but of this there is no trace. He successfully bridged the canyon separating the upper and lower orders of those days, and only hints here and there betray his position above the accepted veterinary station — the witnesses to his will, for example: Isaac Gill and Albert Hutchins, respectively butler and footman at his London residence in Eaton Square.

The last link with the 1844 Charter was broken when James Beart Simonds died. Of the seven signatories, he lived by far the longest, and survived Charles Spooner, the sixth to die, by thirty-three years. He has appeared many times in this tale, for his life was the history of the profession. It is regrettable that for reasons not certainly identified, but possibly personal, Simonds has found little favour with veterinary historian Sir Frederick Smith. Smith's unfounded criticism of Simonds at the time of the cattle plague epidemic of 1865, has already been noted. Apart from acknowledging Simond's ability as an administrator, Smith has repeatedly denigrated the man and his work. Close examination of this antipathy is here impossible, except to recall that Smith was a student at the London school when Simonds was Principal, a special relationship that, then as now, can create feelings of affection, or distaste. There is extensive documentary evidence that Simond's personal contributions to the profession have not been surpassed by any other individual. First a rural practitioner, then Professor of Cattle Pathology at the London school. Member of the Charter Committee and signatory to the Charter. Field investigator of diseases of sheep and cattle, notably sheep-pox, foot-and-mouth disease, pleuro-pneumonia, cattle plague, and parasitic diseases. First veterinary adviser to the Royal Agricultural Society and to the Privy Council. Veterinary adviser to the Privy Council in the successful control of cattle plague, and first veterinary surgeon in the Government department in consequence established. For many years editor-in-chief of *The Veterinarian*. Author of numerous scientific papers. RCVS Councillor for over twenty years, and President in 1862. Principal of the

London school for ten years, and architect of its incorporating Charter of 1875. In retirement, historian and biographer. Because he thought deliberately and spoke quietly, Simonds has been over-shadowed by more flamboyant but less worthy men.

*   *   *

An unpremeditated veterinary revolution began in 1902. In January of that year no one would have forecast that by 1905 several universities would be concerned with veterinary education. At the time it seemed that the veterinary schools — one each in London, Glasgow and Dublin, and two in Edinburgh — were fashioning all the veterinary surgeons, in calibre and number, that the country needed. Only a revolution could change this *status quo*.

Timing of the revolution was precisely right.

It will be recalled that William Dick's will of 1866 made provision for sister Mary, but left the veterinary school in trust to Edinburgh's Town Council. Year after year, the Provost and Councillors of that city struggled to discharge the obligation to maintain Dick's school, but by mid-1902 it had become what *The Edinburgh Evening Dispatch* described as "an embarrassing heritage." At that time the trustees were anxiously wondering how to transplant their responsibilities without breaking faith with William Dick.

Eyes turned to the University, that had just acquired a legacy dating back to the will of William's sister, Mary Dick.

Mary was no ordinary maiden lady. Two years older than her brother, it has been recorded by the late Professor O.C. Bradley that she was "general censor of the manners and morals of the students, and before her had to appear, much to their embarrassment, all delinquents." Not only that, but for several years after her brother's death "she expected the College Principal to visit her every Sunday," to report on the condition and activities of the school. To these indications of iron will, may be added comment from an obituary notice in *The Scotsman* of 1883: "She was an ardent Liberal, and advocated female suffrage; greatly satirical on modern extravagance and effeminacy; boasting, for example, that she had never taken a walk for health in her life, and that she had never had a cough."

She was a wealthy woman, and it was confidently expected that her estate would enhance the finances of the Edinburgh school.

To general astonishment, not so, at least not at that moment, nor for many years to come. Mary Dick's will was as eccentric as her distaste for fresh air. After detailing a number of small legacies, she directed that the residue of her estate should be held in trust "until it amounts to £20,000, when it shall be divided into two equal portions, £10,000 being applied in furtherance of . . . the Veterinary College, and the other £10,000 in the founding of a Professorship either of comparative anatomy or of surgical anatomy . . . in the University of Edinburgh." There was no veterinary surgeon among the trustees. *The Scotsman* commented: "A professorship of this kind in the University will do nothing to advance veterinary medicine and surgery, and it is evident that Miss Dick was not well advised in making this disposition of her property."

Ill-advised she may have been (although it would seem that Mary Dick required advice from no one), but her legacy matured twenty years later, just when it had become clear that a body other than Edinburgh Town Council must accept responsibility for Dick's veterinary school. To the money now available was added £15,000 generously donated by Inglis McCallum, MRCVS, to create a new Administrative Board. *The Veterinary Record* for 20th June 1903 reported: "The University of Edinburgh shall make arrangements under which a degree in veterinary science shall be conferred upon the students of the College who pass the curriculum of the College and attend such classes in the University as may be prescribed. For the purposes of the degree, the College shall be recognised by the University as an extra-mural Veterinary School." At the same time, the University Chair in comparative anatomy envisaged by Mary Dick was to be established, and arrangements made for classes to be held, as convenient, within the university or the veterinary school.

The authorities in Edinburgh had been punctilious in keeping the RCVS informed of these moves, and had emphasised that there was no question of challenging the right of the RCVS to be the only licensing body for the profession. The matter was discussed at length by the RCVS Council on 2nd July 1903; Solicitor Thatcher quoted a letter from the Town Clerk of Edinburgh, acting for the veterinary school: "All candidates should have passed the Royal College examination before being qualified to take the University degree. Thus, there would be no attempt to interfere with the privileges of the Royal College of Veterinary Surgeons; the new degree would be academical only, and additional to the Royal College degree."

This was an exciting new idea, and RCVS Councillor Dollar caught the mood of the moment when he declared: "This scheme . . . has been rendered possible through the munificent bequests of two individuals, the late Professor Dick and his sister, Miss Mary Dick, and by a gentleman who is still living, Mr McCallum . . . we should hail the scheme with enthusiasm, and should support other schools in endeavouring to obtain like advantages."

The timing was absolutely right, because, in a rapidly widening Edwardian world, the profession immediately recognised the scientific and social significance of adding a university degree to a veterinary diploma.

It seemed as if universities throughout the land had been awaiting this moment to enthuse about veterinary education. Discussions started everywhere, some with a *soupçon* of patronage, some with flattery, some with zeal to convert the infidel. The upshot was that by November 1905, *The Veterinary Record* could announce: "In London, Liverpool, Edinburgh and Dublin we now have opportunities of securing University degrees." Add to this, the announcement in May 1904 of a Diploma course in Veterinary State Medicine at the Victoria University of Manchester, and a year later at the University of Cambridge Medical School, a Long Vacation course for "Senior Students, Medical Men and Veterinary Surgeons," and it will be realised that there was now no excuse for uneducated veterinary gentlemen.

Liverpool University provided the only problem for the RCVS in this explosive participation of universities in veterinary education. The university was young in 1904, with a reputation to establish. It had a brash professor, Rubert Boyce, F.R.S., who was determined to make his mark by using the current interest in veterinary education to 'discover' that veterinary surgeons should be trained in universities. This viewpoint was abrasively different from that of Edinburgh University, where it had been tactfully indicated that the veterinary school might, with advantage to all, be related to the University. Boyce addressed meetings, deplored the low level of veterinary education, and averred that if only Liverpool University were given the opportunity to educate veterinary surgeons, what superior fellows they would be. By early 1904 it became known that the University had quietly and successfully negotiated with Principal Owen Williams to take over the New Edinburgh veterinary school, lock, stock, and Sign Manual.

That put the fat right in the RCVS fire, because to co-operate with a university over a degree/diploma course in veterinary science was one thing, but to sanction metamorphosis into a university faculty of an entire school affiliated to the RCVS was very much another.

Had Williams, Boyce and the Liverpool University authorities been less secretive, the RCVS would have been less suspicious of their motives. It was strongly suspected that they hoped to establish not only a teaching, but also a licensing school. This, however, was denied.

The proposed transfer of the New Edinburgh school to Liverpool was first discussed by the RCVS at a meeting on 8th April 1904, during the course of which it became clear that negotiations were well advanced; indeed, the buildings in Edinburgh were already advertised for sale. It happened that the Principal of the New Edinburgh school, Owen Williams, was also President of the RCVS, and more than one Councillor felt that he could have been more forthcoming with his colleagues. Indeed, an item to be considered at that meeting was a letter dated 10th February from the Home Office, seeking Council's observations on "an application from Mr W. Owen Williams for permission to remove the New Veterinary College, Edinburgh, as a teaching establishment from Edinburgh to Liverpool." This letter had been acknowledged by Williams as RCVS President, with the promise that it would be put to the Council at the next quarterly meeting on 8th April, but some Councillors felt that they should have had an earlier opportunity to reply.

There was distrust and irritation in the discussions about Liverpool, in contrast to the friendly negotiations with Edinburgh. Finally there was blunt opposition by the body of the RCVS, and a reply to the Home Office expressing "disapproval of the proposal to establish a second Veterinary College in England."

RCVS Solicitor Thatcher was asked to determine "the nature of the privileges conferred by affiliation to the Royal College of Veterinary Surgeons, and . . . whether these privileges can be disposed of by sale or otherwise without the consent of the Council." His report was presented to the Council on 22nd April 1904, and concluded that as far as the New Edinburgh school was concerned, "I do not think that the Royal College of Veterinary Surgeons has any voice in the matter."

So that was that.

The New Edinburgh school was closed in the latter part of 1904, to reappear as the Veterinary Faculty of the University of Liverpool. It was a teaching school only, however, and its students had to take RCVS examinations. Owen Williams became Professor of the Principles and Practice of Veterinary Medicine and Surgery.

*   *   *

Important though education of the profession might be, and momentous its new relationship with universities, these were matters for a handful of veterinary academics. Most veterinary surgeons in the early twentieth century had still to be more concerned with today's bread than with tomorrow's cake, and it was by no means clear where a living was to be found in the years immediately ahead. Certainly, the time was long past when a veterinary surgeon was expected merely to treat an animal and charge a fee; cattle plague left that world behind in 1865, for the concept was then born of prevention as well as control of animal diseases. The bacteriological discoveries of the last two decades of the nineteenth century, had stretched the horizon of infectious diseases apparently to infinity, with new veterinary roles to be played. But until the turn of the century these were occupations for a few, for there was little official backing (i.e. money) for extensive disease control.

The Diamond Jubilee approached with the puff and splutter of the horseless carriage, of which a *Veterinary Record* editorial of 4th July 1896 tried to forecast the veterinary significance. On balance, there was reassurance for those "who are considering the possibilities of the veterinary profession as a means of livelihood, to put aside the downfall of the horse as an item likely to affect their chances."

True, the take-over of power without horses came more slowly than some had anticipated. In 1904, for example, the London General Omnibus Company were still deeply concerned about glanders in their stables, and obtained RCVS cooperation in discussing the matter with representatives of London horse-owners possessing some 145,000 animals. However, the electric tram and the motor-car *were* coming, and horses *were* disappearing, and it behoved a veterinary son to be prepared in 1905 *not* to do as Dad had done.

CHAPTER 14

John McFadyean — leader of the profession

Something has been said of John McFadyean's exceptional academic training, of his skill as a scientific investigator, especially as a microscopist, of his success as teacher and administrator, and of the impact of his *Journal of Comparative Pathology and Therapeutics*. The circumstances have been described of his move to London in 1892, to be Dean and Professor of Pathology and Bacteriology at the London school, where one of his first concerns was to organise the laboratory that had been established with part of the annual grant from the Royal Agricultural Society. In this he was so successful that by the time he was promoted Principal in 1894, the laboratory was known throughout the profession as willing to give practical help and sound advice. That laboratory was the first in Britain devoted exclusively to veterinary diagnosis and research.

McFadyean was elected to the Council of the RCVS in 1893, and took an active part in its affairs.

Thus, by 1894 McFadyean was Principal of the oldest and largest British veterinary school. He was the most experienced veterinary pathologist in the country, personally directing a unique laboratory. He owned and edited one of the world's outstanding veterinary research journals, and he was privy to the deliberations of the ruling Council of the profession. In short, at forty-one he was among the leaders of his people.

The list of McFadyean's scientific reports and original publications during the decade following his move to London, reads like the index to a text-book on pathology. If the papers did not actually exist (to be read, and re-read, with profit three generations later), it would be excusable to doubt that a single individual could produce such a mass of original material. Fleming was a prodigious writer, but far less was creative than was copied. There have been others who have written expansively and well, but no one has approached McFadyean in quantity of observational research of the highest quality. He was not a theoretician, however — no

John Gamgee. Indeed, his few creative attempts were unconvincing, and he wisely (or instinctively) left that field to others. But as an observer, and recorder of what he saw, he stands supreme.

It would be tedious even to summarise McFadyean's researches during this period, but two episodes are historically important. One concerns African Horse-sickness, the other tuberculosis.

African Horse-sickness is a highly lethal disease, of cause unknown in 1899, but postulated by investigators in South Africa to be a fungus. McFadyean became involved with African Horse-sickness through one of those bizarre incidents that are the stuff of scientific discovery.

The bacteriological revolution, dating from 1882, demonstrated a range of micro-organisms as the cause of diseases such as tuberculosis, glanders, anthrax, tetanus. After several years of successfully linking one infectious disease after another with a micro-organism that could be seen under the microscope, and grown in the laboratory, an enigma was noticed in every bacteriological laboratory. Certain highly infectious diseases, such as foot-and-mouth disease, rabies, and cattle plague, did not appear to be associated with a micro-organism. Try as scientists would — and they tried in their dozens — nothing could be seen under the microscope, and nothing grew in laboratory culture from animals killed by these diseases.

The mystery was accidentally solved by the Germans Fredrich Loeffler and Paul Frosch. In trying to purify fluid from the vesicles that are characteristic of foot-and-mouth disease, these workers filtered it through unglazed porcelain with pores too fine to allow passage of bacteria. To their astonishment, they found that this bacteria-free filtrate still produced foot-and-mouth disease when injected into cattle. They confirmed this observation several times, realised its significance, and focussed world attention on a hitherto unsuspected class of pathogenic micro-organisms, the so-called ultra-visible viruses. Thus was born the science of virology, as important, and as vast, as its predecessor bacteriology.

This discovery was published in 1898, and McFadyean was one of a small number of British veterinarians — perhaps the only one — to read the original paper. He translated and summarised it, and published it in the first number of his *Journal* for 1899.

Enter African Horse-sickness.

McFadyean acquired a few unglazed porcelain filters of the kind used by Loeffler and Frosch, and shortly afterwards was given for laboratory examination a bottle of blood that William Robertson (back in Britain from the Bacteriological Institute at the Cape of Good Hope) had taken in South Africa from a horse that had died of African Horse-sickness. On

13th October 1899 McFadyean injected this blood into a horse. Eight days later it died of African Horse-sickness. He repeated the observation with the same result. Then he took blood and pericandial fluid from an experimental case of the disease, mixed them, and passed the mixture through a filter of unglazed porcelain. On 9th December 1899 he injected this filtrate into another horse. Eight days later, it too died of African Horse-sickness.

In this manner McFadyean identified a second animal disease caused by an ultra-visible virus. Virologists will recognise the odds against success in thus demonstrating a virus disease, and no one can be unimpressed by the coincidence that the one veterinary pathologist in Britain in possession of a few unglazed porcelain filters, and with the technical ability to use them, had been presented with material containing a virus tough enough to survive a sea voyage from South Africa. No matter. Gods play the odds, and sometimes win.

The historically important tuberculosis episode involving McFadyean was far removed from sick horses in the stables of the London veterinary school. It was, in fact, a difference of opinion between John McFadyean and Robert Koch, publicly expressed at the International Tuberculosis Congress held in London in July 1901.

McFadyean's special knowledge of tuberculosis in animals, dating back to studies in the 1880's, was recognised by an invitation to present one of only three papers to be given in plenary session at the Congress. Robert Koch had agreed to give the first of these, on combating tuberculosis. The next day, Frenchman Brouardel would speak on Public Health aspects of the disease. On the third afternoon, McFadyean would present a paper on: "Danger to Man of Milk from Tuberculous Cows."

The Congress, with some 2,500 delegates, was under Royal and noble patronage. The world-wide significance of tuberculosis at that time, in Man and animals, may be gauged from two statistics presented at the Congress. In Germany at that moment, 226,000 persons over the age of fifteen were in hospital with tuberculosis. In Britain thirty per cent of dairy cattle were tuberculous, and two per cent of these were excreting tubercle bacilli in their milk.

Lord Lister was chairman for Koch's address, and there was an immense audience. Koch's theme was that measures to control diseases must be related to the characteristics of those diseases. Thus, rabies in Man is prevented by destroying rabid animals; cholera is controlled by dealing with contaminated water, and so on. Then he asked rhetorically if the most rational methods were being used to combat tuberculosis? He thought not. Too much importance, he contended, was attached to the hazard for Man of contact with tuberculous animals. He then made two statements that well-nigh pole-axed his audience. First: "Human tuberculosis differs from bovine and cannot be transmitted to cattle." Secondly: "I should estimate the extent of infection by the milk and flesh of tubercular cattle, and butter made from their milk, as hardly greater than hereditary transmission, and I therefore do not deem it advisable to take any measures against it."

These conclusions contradicted the beliefs of virtually every medical man and veterinary surgeon in the audience, and caused a sensation. Chairman Lord Lister referred to: "The startling thesis that bovine tuberculosis is incapable of development in man."

Nobody envied McFadyean the task of trying to persuade the same audience, two days later, that milk from tuberculous cattle was dangerous. The Master had declared the matter unimportant. Those who thought McFadyean might compromise were vastly wrong. He said: "The greatest living authority on tuberculosis- — the world renowned discoverer of the tubercle bacillus, and the man to whom we are mainly indebted for our knowledge of the cause of tuberculosis — has declared his conviction that human and bovine tuberculosis are practically distinct diseases. I do not know how far the reasons assigned by Dr Koch for the opinion he now holds on this question may have commended themselves to the members of the Congress, but I am overwhelmed to find myself in a position which compels me to offer some criticism on the pronouncement of one the latchet of whose shoes I am not worthy to unloose."

He then disagreed with Koch, absolutely, saying, amongst many things: "The almost entire absence of any law dealing with tuberculous udder disease in cows is a scandal and reproach to civilisation."

No matter what McFadyean said, of course, Koch's reputation was such that his opinions could not be ignored. Medical and veterinary men were grateful to McFadyean for so deftly and courageously staking his reputation to disagree with Koch on a world-wide stage, but discovery of the truth was so important that it must be established at the earliest possible moment.

Experiments to test Koch's statements were initiated in many countries. In Britain, a Royal Commission under the chairmanship of Sir Michael Foster, with McFadyean a member, was set up within weeks. Its terms of reference were to determine whether tuberculosis in animals was the same disease as in Man, and whether it was communicable from Man to animals and from animals to Man.

Most Royal Commissions reach conclusions by collecting and collating data supplied by experts in the field under review. In this case, however, the brief was to examine the validity of statements made by the world's greatest authority on the subject. The members of the Commission were forced, therefore, to design and prosecute their own experiments. It was a formidable undertaking, especially as many observations had to be made on cattle. There was no Governmental provision for medical or veterinary research on that scale. Fortunately, however, Sir James Blyth generously made available two small farms near Stansted in Essex, and a house in the village. There, over the next ten years, with McFadyean always deeply involved, classic experiments were carried out that were described in the Commission's Reports of 1904, 1907, 1909 and 1911. In the fullness of time, McFadyean's views were amply vindicated.

The significance of the Koch/McFadyean episode was that it emphasised the specialist help that veterinary surgeons could give in the field of Public Health, and that it drew urgent attention to the need for Government support for research on animal diseases.

John McFadyean was knighted in 1905, in recognition of his services to veterinary science and agriculture, with special reference to the Royal Commission on Tuberculosis. The news was hailed with delight that has not been equalled, and six hundred and twenty-nine veterinary surgeons (approximately one fifth of the profession) subscribed to a splendid presentation to the man whom they recognised as their leader.

It was on McFadyean's recommendation to Lord Onslow, President of the Board of Agriculture and Fisheries, that the historically important appointment was made in April 1904 of Stewart Stockman to be Chief Veterinary Officer, with effect from 1st January 1905. This was in succession to Alexander Cope, retiring after many years of devoted service to the Veterinary Department.

It will be recalled that Stockman had volunteered in 1900 for service in the Boer War. When hostilities ended, he worked for a year in the Indian Civil Veterinary Department, then returned to South Africa as Principal Veterinary Officer in the Transvaal. He was in South Africa when invited to be Chief Veterinary Officer in Britain. McFadyean had known Stockman as one of his students at the Edinburgh veterinary school, and as his successor there as teacher of pathology and bacteriology. Stockman had published several papers in McFadyean's *Journal*, and their relationship was of colleagues, rather than of professor and pupil. There was no favouritism in the appointment, because although only thirty-five years old, Stockman was, by character and training, the best man available, but it was a happy coincidence that the two were close friends. In 1908 friendship blossomed into a family relationship, when Stewart Stockman married Elizabeth Ethel, McFadyean's older daughter.

Intimate professional and personal contact between McFadyean and Stockman, who shared the highest academic, scientific, Governmental and political positions, profoundly influenced development of the veterinary profession for two decades.

*   *   *

Poor health forced RCVS Secretary Arthur W. Hill to resign in 1906: "I have been advised to give up so great a responsibility." At a meeting of the RCVS Council on 5th October this resignation was accepted. The President thanked Hill, who "for the long period of twenty-seven years . . . has faithfully and to the best of his abilities discharged the duties of Secretary . . . the Council has resolved to award you a pension during the remainder of your life of £40 per annum." Many members of the profession contributed to a farewell gift to this kindly and courteous man.

Advertisements were immediately placed in *The Times*, *The Telegraph*, *The Veterinary Record*, and *Law Times*: "Secretary to the Royal College of Veterinary Surgeons. Salary £250 per annum. Age not to exceed 40 years . . ." Some one hundred applications were received. On 4th January 1907 Messers Bullock, Sydenham and Smith were "severally and searchingly interviewed, and ultimately it was decided to recommend Mr Bullock." Bullock was called before the Council, informed that he had been selected, and said: "I shall always do my best so to serve you that you will never regret the choice you have made today." His duties as Secretary began on 1st February 1907.

Within a few weeks it was clear that the RCVS had acquired in Fred Bullock an exceptional person. He immediately recognised that the Register was a travesty of the accurate professional muster-book it ought to be. The 1881 Veterinary Surgeon's Act made the Register the cornerstone of the profession. It was to be accepted as evidence in courts of law. Registered men were veterinary surgeons (or 'Registered Practitioners'), and men whose names were not in the Register could not call themselves veterinary surgeons. Yet for some twenty-five years, Secretary Hill, and various Presidents and Councillors, had made no serious attempt to keep the Register up-to-date. It was an odd oversight for people who could be pernickety about procedure at meetings, and censorious of other administrative shortcomings.

Bullock set about revising the Register, and was praised by *The Veterinary Record* of 7th March 1908: "Mr Bullock has earned the gratitude of the profession for his first year's work as Registrar." The legal obligation of the Register to provide "an accurate list of our members" was emphasised, and it was noted that over 700 alterations of addresses had been necessary out of a total of some 3,400 names. In particular, scrutiny had reduced the number of Registered Practitioners, by death, from over 400 to 319. There was commendation, too, for "a serious attempt . . . throughout the volume to facilitate its use," and for "a detailed index, in addition to the table of contents." Succeeding years brought further improvements, and the accuracy of the Register was never again in doubt.

* * *

Veterinary surgeon Francis Whitfield Wragg, practitioner of London, died in 1908. He gave much to the profession, as RCVS Councillor and Treasurer for many years, and as President in 1893. In paying tribute, *The Veterinary Record* of 22nd August 1908 noted especially his influence as a member of the Council of the Royal Society for the Prevention of Cruelty to Animals (RSPCA), in improving relations between that body and the veterinary profession. The *Record* commented: "Theoretically, the Society and the profession have a common aim . . . the two bodies might be expected to work in unison; but we all know that this is far from being the case."

The RSPCA was formed in 1824, and from its earliest days there were cordial relations with many individual veterinary surgeons. Charles Spooner, Principal of the London school from 1853 to 1871, for example, was deeply interested in the Society, and Edmund Gabriel, first Secretary of the RCVS, was elected in 1856 to be its veterinary surgeon. In 1908, however, at the level of the profession itself, as distinct from individuals within it, relations were cool and sometimes hostile.

Veterinary surgeons did not question the need to control cruelty to animals, and the insensitivity of earlier times was excused by no one. Indeed, the brutality of experimental exploitation of animals in Europe in the 18th and early 19th centuries was too sickening to contemplate, and the RSPCA deserved credit for controlling it. Cruelty to animals was indefinable, however, and attitudes varied widely. Differences between the RSPCA and the veterinary profession were almost always over cases of so-called cruelty that were an expression of opinion, not of clear-cut fact. Three additional factors increased tension. First, many leading figures in the RSPCA were aristocrats, with a tendency to impose their will and to patronise. Secondly the Society was wealthy and uninhibited about taking legal action. Thirdly, with rare exceptions, the Society's inspectors had no special knowledge of animals.

Small wonder, therefore, that cases against veterinary surgeons brought to the courts by the RSPCA (and they were by no means uncommon), caused professional offence. An example will make the point. At the RCVS Annual General Meeting in May 1892, Mr A. Leather said: "I should like to draw the attention of the meeting and the Council in particular to prosecutions that have taken place against members of the profession. It appears to me . . . that the Society for the Prevention of Cruelty to Animals are trying to get the upper hand of the profession." To this comment, Mr W. Woods added: "A member of the profession had under his treatment a horse. At the end of nine days he gave it as his opinion that the horse was fit for light work . . . the owner was summoned by the Society for the Prevention of Cruelty to Animals, and the veterinary surgeon was also summoned for cruelty . . . is it legal . . . for a veterinary surgeon to be summoned in a criminal court?"

*   *   *

"Injured Animals in London" was the subject of a *Veterinary Record* editorial in April 1906, emphasising the unsatisfactory arrangements for humane and expeditious destruction of badly injured horses: "The duty of the police is to call in the nearest veterinary surgeon . . . when the advice is . . . slaughter . . . the next step is to obtain a horse-slaughterer. There are six knackers' yards in the metropolis, but all are removed from the centre of the town . . . there would be no difficulty . . . if the police were on the Telephone Exchange. They are not, but trust to their own telegraph wires connecting the different stations . . . a constable, having secured a veterinary certificate for slaughter, has to go to the nearest police station and wire to the one nearest to a knacker's. From there a constable walks to the knacker's and probably finds no man disengaged. If the police used the telephone they could communicate direct with all the knackers and receive an immediate reply."

That conundrum was reduced to insignificance, however, without recourse to the telephone.

Five months later another *Veterinary Record* editorial noted the beginning of the solution to the problem. There were "about 600 motor-buses now running in London . . . the . . . horse-drawn omnibuses cannot compete with a motor. People like the novelty and wait for it. They like to travel fast . . . the noise, stink and dust . . . are left behind" for others.

By 1908 there was serious hardship among those who had lived by horses. *The Daily Telegraph* noted that: "The London Road Car Company is . . . shortly disposing of stabling and other premises" for "about 800 horses," with consequent loss of employment for stablemen, hay and corn merchants, farriers, harness-makers, and veterinary surgeons. In the same year, the Metropolitan Police Commissioner's report for numbers of buses and trams, showed horse-drawn vehicles down by 908, and mechanical up by 794. *The Yorkshire Post* said in January 1910: "During the Christmas week there was an immense sale of hansom cabs and horses in London . . . no great demand . . . prices . . . trifling . . . a leading firm of cab-owners predicted that within two years hardly a hansom cab would be seen . . . in London." In August 1911 *The Veterinary Record* reported: "The London General Omnibus Company are selling off horses at the rate of 100 a week, and expect by the end of next month to have taken off the road their remaining 94 horse-omnibuses."

That was August. Two months later the same journal carried a letter from Henry Taylor of Hayward's Heath, beginning: "A motor car has become such a necessary adjunct to a veterinary practice in these days of rapid transit that a short summary of what the annual cost of a small car amounts to would probably interest many of your readers. Mine is an 8 h.p. Renault two-seater . . ." Mr Taylor was right. Several letters followed, covering a 6 h.p. Rover, a 7 to 9 h.p. Swift, another 6 h.p. Rover, an 8 h.p. Rover, and a 12 h.p. Delage. Cost per mile was about sixpence (including, of course, the chauffeur's wages).

*   *   *

The National Veterinary School of Lyons in France, the oldest veterinary school in the world, celebrated its one hundred and fiftieth anniversary in 1912. An invitation was received by the RCVS to send delegates to the celebrations. At a meeting of the Council on 11th October, President Mettam, Principal of the Dublin veterinary school, said: "I understand that Sir John McFadyean and Mr Stockman will be in Lyons . . . and I myself am also intending to visit Lyons on the same occasion. Perhaps the College might see fit to delegate Sir John McFadyean, Mr Stockman, and myself as representatives of the College on this occasion."

A resolution in favour was enthusiastically proposed by Councillor Trigger, and seconded by Councillor Lawson. It was "carried with acclamation."

Who could better represent the RCVS than John McFadyean and two of his pupils of Edinburgh days, now the three most influential men in the British veterinary profession?

CHAPTER 15

A veterinary diploma in Public Health. A registration fee

The one hundred and fiftieth anniversary celebrations at the Lyons veterinary school in the autumn of 1912, attracted veterinary surgeons from many countries, but especially from the European nations where veterinary education was born. All was friendliness and reminiscence. French and Germans and Belgians and Russians and Austrians and British. Who would have foretold the holocaust ahead? As with all twentieth century history, veterinary events are located before, during, after, or between the First and Second World Wars, in the context of the political, social, and material consequences of those convulsions.

One of London's great monuments was completed in the summer of 1912, ahead of the First War, and unscathed by bombs in the Second. The huge Quadriga of Peace, all of forty tons, sixty feet above the ground, astride Decimus Burton's Arch at the top of Constitution Hill: war horses reined back by a startled charioteer, as the angel Peace alights beside him. It is always splendid, but truly magnificent floating above leafless trees against the hard sky of a winter's afternoon, seen to greatest advantage looking east from Grosvenor Crescent, that joins Grosvenor Place to Belgrave Square.

Belgrave Square is now the home of the Royal College of Veterinary Surgeons. The sculptor of the Quadriga of Peace was veterinary surgeon Adrian Jones.

Alfred Adrian Jones was born in Ludlow in 1845 into a family 'in easy circumstances.' Father James Brookhandling Jones was "a keen horseman . . . able to mount us all, so that very early in our 'teens we could follow the Ludlow Foxhounds." Adrian found fisticuffs, ratting, rabbiting and horses more congenial than the curriculum at Ludlow Grammar School, with the single exception of a drawing class on Monday afternoons. It was "a shock when this easy time came to an end, and my father told me that I was to become a veterinary surgeon. This was a sort of compromise. I disliked the idea of business and he disliked the idea of art and if I had to take a profession, one that brought me into contact with horses was the most agreeable."

Adrian Jones received his MRCVS diploma from the London veterinary school in April 1865, joined the Army and was gazetted veterinary surgeon to the Royal Horse Artillery in India. Horses were his life, riding and racing them, and training them for brother officers. He served in the Abyssinian campaign of 1868, returned briefly to India, then back to England to join the Queen's Bays. Next ten years in Ireland, recalling in old age: "That decade was the pleasantest of my life; chiefly on account of the sport — the hunting and steeple-chasing." He was with the 7th Hussars during the Boer War of 1881, then returned to England, being quartered in London, where "for the first time I entered the world of artists." During these Army years he had been painting compulsively in every spare moment — horses, horses, horses. He was essentially untutored, and his splendid talent was eyed askance by conservative Academicians who believed that legitimate artists must attend conventional schools.

He was befriended, however, by Charles Bell Birch, A.R.A., who, recognising exceptional natural ability and professional understanding of animal anatomy, encouraged him to take up sculpture, and taught him all he knew. That Birch's instinct was correct was proved when one of Jones's first pieces, a statuette of one of his own hunters, was exhibited at the Royal Academy in 1884.

This artistic interlude was interrupted by the Nile Expedition, with Jones veterinary surgeon to the Camel Corps, and he was thus engaged when he heard that the London Goldsmith's Company had awarded him first prize for a statuette of a huntsman with two hounds, titled "Gone Away."

After twenty-three years' service, he abandoned the Army for fulltime painting and sculpture, and received more commissions than he could fulfil. Virtually all his work centred on horses, and included many famous names of the day.

A prototype of the eventual Quadriga of Peace, exhibited by Jones at the Royal Academy of 1891, caught the eye of the Prince of Wales, who sent for the sculptor. "He made a proposal that filled me with astonishment and pleasure. This was that the Arch on the top of Constitution Hill . . . would make an ideal site for a Quadriga to be founded on the one he had admired at Burlington House." The Prince suggested that drawings be submitted to the Office of Works. Annually, for the next sixteen years, Jones was informed by that Office that the project was not forgotten, but could not be implemented for lack of funds. Then, out of nowhere, Lord Michelham agreed to foot the bill, and work began in 1907.

The former Prince of Wales, now King Edward VII, was greatly interested in the development of his idea, and frequently visited Jones's studio. The magnitude of the undertaking fascinated him. The armature for each horse, for example, weighed two tons, to be buried in seven tons of clay; the chariot was nine feet by eighteen, with wheels eight feet across. "My studio was only big enough to carry out the construction of one item of the group in turn, and . . . I could never see the completed whole until . . . every piece had been cast in bronze."

The bronze casting was carried out by A.B. Burton of Thames Ditton. His problems, too, were vast, not the least being transportation of huge plaster casts to the foundry, and of the bronzes back to Constitution Hill. Reinforcement of the Arch was a saga on its own.

King Edward died two years before the work was finished. Adrian Jones had hoped for (and had planned) a memorable unveiling ceremony. Officialdom decreed otherwise. There was no ceremony. A plaque records the munificence of Lord Michelham. Reward for Adrian Jones is in the joy of generations.

                    *   *   *

A Supplementary Charter was granted to the RCVS just after the outbreak of war in 1914. The decision to apply for a Charter had been taken at a meeting of the Council in July 1913, and a draft was approved three months later. The purpose of the first clause was to alter the date of the Annual General Meeting from the first Wednesday in June to "any of the first seven days in the month of June." There was more behind this suggestion than the words indicate. By the original Charter of 1844, the Annual General Meeting was to be held in May, but this was changed by the Charter of 1892 to the first Wednesday in June. By an astonishing oversight — in the veterinary, of all professions — it was forgotten that the first Wednesday in June is Derby Day. So for many, over several years, duty to attend the RCVS Annual General Meeting struggled with the lure of Epsom Downs. Hence seizure of this opportunity to see sanity restored.

The second clause reduced the number of Vice-presidents from six to two, as proposed by William Hunting for the Charter of 1892, but overruled at that time. This amendment was overdue, for, as Councillor Clarkson commented: "If we have only two Vice-presidents it will be something more of an honourable position than it is at present with six, and when we practically hawk the post about." The third was a minor clause, reducing from twenty-five years to twenty-three the age at which the Fellowship examination might be taken.

The essential reason for a new Charter was in clause four: "That the Council . . . shall have power to institute a Diploma in Veterinary State Medicine." At that time the RCVS granted only Membership and Fellowship diplomas. The proposal for an additional qualification recognised the rapidly expanding involvement of veterinary surgeons in Public Health, Local Government, and the Veterinary Department of the Board of Agriculture and Fisheries. The decision to seek a new Charter to implement the proposal was the culmination of discussions stretching back to January 1899, when Professor W.O. Williams of the New Edinburgh School (son of its founder) had moved in Council: "That powers be obtained . . . to grant an additional degree to members of the Royal College of Veterinary Surgeons, to be known as that of 'Veterinary Officer of Health.' " Williams emphasised the need to develop veterinary expertise in preventive medicine, and envisaged that candidates for the proposed qualification would receive special instruction on Public Health legislation, infectious diseases, meat inspection, and chemical and bacteriological techniques. His motion was strongly supported by the Chief Veterinary Officer, Councillor Cope.

Councillor McFadyean opposed the motion with characteristic bluntness: "I can hardly imagine anything that is calculated to do the veterinary profession more harm . . . it . . . amounts to this, that the diploma which we at present grant is not a guarantee that the veterinary surgeon is . . . fitted to undertake veterinary duties, including inspection of meat and animals . . . and that the training on which that diploma has been granted is inadequate."

This absolute opposition from the hard-headed McFadyean, reflects the strife at that time between medical and veterinary men over definition of areas of interest of the two professions in the new field of Public Health. Medical men were thrusting for all the senior posts, positive of their superior competence, even in dairy and meat inspection. McFadyean's opinion was that Public Health instruction in veterinary schools should be so comprehensive, that the adequacy of graduates holding only the MRCVS qualification could not be challenged. He was emphatic, however, that veterinary surgeons should confine themselves to veterinary problems.

When Williams's motion was tested, only three of twenty-three Councillors voted in favour. To some extent this may have reflected McFadyean's dominating personality, but his point of view was supported in *The Veterinary Record* by Editor Hunting, whom no one dominated: "The recently educated veterinary surgeon is infinitely the superior of any other person for all duties embraced by veterinary public health."

Six years passed before the subject again came before the RCVS. A committee formed specifically to look into the matter reported in January 1905: "After very careful consideration . . . the time has not yet arrived for recommending the Council to obtain a new Charter in order to institute a Diploma in Veterinary State Medicine." It will be recalled that this was the period of avid interest of universities in veterinary education, with Liverpool and Manchester particularly concerned with veterinary hygiene.

Four years on, and again Owen Williams (now at Liverpool) pressed the RCVS to take interest in a specialist qualification in "State and Municipal Hygiene and Medicine." On this occasion — April 1909 — the Council agreed that a committee should consider "the advisability of granting a diploma." An editorial in *The Veterinary Record* supported reassessment of the problem, because: "The demand for veterinary surgeons to engage in Public Health work has increased . . . it is now recognised that among the many duties . . . some are best performed by medical men, and others by veterinarians . . . such work requires a special training in certain subjects." The committee reported in October 1909, and Council accepted that: "A diploma or certificate in State and Municipal Hygiene and Medicine is desirable." However, the unsatisfactory state of RCVS finances at the time caused the matter, with regret, to be shelved.

As already noted, the decision to apply for a new Charter to cover a Diploma in Veterinary State Medicine was eventually taken in 1913. The Charter was granted in August of the following year. It is a measure of the advance in importance of veterinary involvement in Public Health, that the money required for this Charter was approved in spite of financial difficulties far more serious than those of 1909. Work began immediately on formulating regulations for the new diploma, and these were published in the minutes of the RCVS Council meeting for 8th January 1915. It was decided that candidates must be Members of the RCVS, and, for six months, have received instruction at an affiliated school in epizootiology, veterinary hygiene and toxicology, veterinary bacteriology and protozoology, and chemistry as applied to veterinary hygiene, and "during a separate period of six months . . . have been diligently engaged in acquiring a knowledge of the duties of Veterinary Inspection in the administration of a State Department, County Council, Municipality, or Urban Authority employing one or more whole-time veterinary officers." Written and oral examinations would be held "at a centre of veterinary teaching."

However, worsening fortunes in the war, and the by now alarming financial position of the RCVS made it impossible to implement this first, historic decision on specialist veterinary education. In October 1915 the Council had no option but to decide that it be held "in abeyance until further notice." William Owen Williams died in 1911, long before the first Diploma in Veterinary State Medicine was granted in 1920. His is the credit, however, for envisaging, two decades earlier, that the veterinary role in Public Health would become too specialised to be covered adequately by undergraduate instruction.

* * *

Mention has been made of the precarious financial position of the RCVS in 1915. For sixty years after the 1844 Charter, the RCVS was apparently disinterested in its finances. In 1846 minor expenses associated with Charter were still outstanding, and a circular was "sent to each member of the profession, requesting a yearly subscription of not less than 10s. in support of the Royal College of Veterinary Surgeons," but by 1850 all debts had been paid, and the need for an annual subscription had passed. The only income was from examination fees which covered payment of examiners, rates, and the modest emoluments of the Secretary and caretaker. No effort was made to accumulate capital against exigency. Councillors received no expenses, and it was many years before the principle was accepted that the President should be reimbursed for representing the RCVS on official occasions.

It might have been supposed that shortage of money in the early 1880's, when the RCVS was seeking premises to replace the disintegrating property in Red Lion Square, would have stimulated efforts to create a more substantial financial background for the future, perhaps by introducing an annual registration fee. However, at this time 'Existing Practitioners' were being taken on to the Register under the terms of the 1881 Veterinary Surgeons' Act, and their fees caused a sudden, albeit temporary, increase in income that made a general subscription seem unnecessary. For several years thereafter there was a feeling that the capital thus acquired was adequate, and when the Charter of 1892 was being prepared a clause in the draft, "That there be a registration of 5/ — annually," was unanimously removed.

By the turn of the century, however, finance was causing anxiety, and "unless the examination expenses were very much reduced the financial condition of the College would be considerably embarrassed." In a letter dated 25th May 1901 to *The Veterinary Record*, practitioner Henry Gray urged that: "If every man practising veterinary surgery . . . were called upon to pay an annual registration fee of one guinea" sufficient would be acquired "to enable the RCVS to decently maintain itself." Thus began a nineteen-year marathon over the roughest of roads, to the seemingly simplest of goals — a mandatory registration fee.

On 3rd July 1902 the RCVS Council discussed acquisition of powers to impose a registration fee, and Solicitor Thatcher made it clear that "a fresh Act of Parliament" would be required. He forecast the possibility of opposition from "a great number of the profession," and the certainty of paying "a good lot of money." Reflecting on this opinion, Council tried to forget the matter. However, it was brought back to their consciousness in July 1906 (with John McFadyean recently elected President) by a resolution from the Central Veterinary Medical Association suggesting imposition of a registration fee. Adopting the classic first line of defence, the matter was referred to a committee, which, three months later, advised against the idea as "they had no evidence that the majority of the profession . . . would consent to be taxed in the way suggested."

McFadyean was re-elected President in July 1907, and at the next meeting introduced the item: "Annual Registration fee. To consider the advisability of taking the opinion of the profession on this matter." The profession was indeed consulted, and of those who replied to a questionnaire, 1234 were in favour and 376 were against an annual registration fee. On the basis of this referendum, the Council decided to apply for an Act to amend the 1881 Veterinary Surgeons' Act. There was speedy action, with a draft Bill by October 1907. Most of this was concerned with the registration fee, but collective enthusiasm unwisely included a clause "extending the powers of the R.C.V.S. with regard to quackery." It would be an offence for anyone not entitled to call himself a veterinary surgeon, to "recover in any Court any fee . . . for performing any Veterinary operation, or for giving any Veterinary attendance or advice or for acting in any manner as a Veterinary Surgeon."

Unhappily, what the RCVS intended as additional protection for the public against unskilled treatment, was seen outside the profession as a sly attempt to provide extra employment for veterinary surgeons, by preventing shepherds from castrating lambs, herdsmen from calving cows, and any custodian of animals from carrying out similar simple acts of husbandry. Of course the RCVS had no intention of curtailing these time-honoured duties, but once the contents of the Bill were known the damage was done. The agricultural community was in highest dudgeon, and swore opposition to the death. Members of the Highland and Agricultural Society were particularly incensed, and comment from the

National Sheep Breeders' Association was: "It is practically a Veterinary Surgeons Emolument Bill."

That was the outside opposition. Within the profession, passions raged unchecked. Those who had voted against the registration fee turned out to be minor in numbers, but major in voice. They were led by RCVS Councillors J.A.W. Dollar, W.F. Barrett and J.R.U. Dewar, with rank-and-file support organised by J.S. Hurndall. The objections were that the RCVS did not require so large an annual income, and that it was heinous to remove a man's name from the Register for non-payment of a paltry annual guinea. In the manner of parochial crusaders, this minority alleged that there would be rule by bludgeon and that individual liberty was at stake.

Hurndall, Honorary Secretary to the "Grand Committee organised to oppose the proposed Veterinary Surgeons' Act (1881) Amendment Bill," submitted to the Privy Council a petition dated 29th April 1909, signed by "880 Fellows and Members of the Royal College of Veterinary Surgeons." Their Lordships were assured that "the interests of the veterinary profession will best be served by not lending support to further prosecution of the measure."

This document must be among the most trivial, yet most damaging, submitted to the Privy Council by a minority indicting a majority in the same profession. The prospect of an assured income for the RCVS was destroyed for years.

Meanwhile, in spite of rigorous economies, RCVS expenditure continued to exceed income, and every year withdrawal of capital was unavoidable. The outbreak of war in 1914 brought a sudden drop in numbers of students, and their examination fees were lost. By April 1915 there was a bank overdraft, and Treasurer Mulvey was in "conversation with the bank manager," who was becoming restive about lack of security to cover increasing borrowing. There was talk of depositing with the bank the deeds of No. 10 Red Lion Square. On 5th June 1915 *The Veterinary Record* said: "We may yet be forced to save the College from bankruptcy by a voluntary subscription — while we await the passage of the Bill." A plea to the Treasury for a special grant was, with regret, refused and at the Council meeting of 2nd July 1915, a desperate Treasurer Mulvey asked: "Where is the money to come from?" In reply, there were: "Cries of, 'The profession' and 'The Bill.' " It was explained to those not already aware of the decision, that the Bill had been abandoned until the war was over. The only hope now was that the profession, as individuals, would save their ruling body. Not everyone was in favour of begging, but *The Veterinary Record* strongly supported the appeal. The suggested donation was one guinea annually until the Bill was achieved. There were many sympathetic ears, and by 1918 this voluntary income topped £1000 a year.

The Veterinary Surgeons' Act (1881) Amendment Act, permitting the RCVS to impose a registration fee and thus acquire an annual income, reached the Statute Book in August 1920.

*   *   *

William Hunting, founder in 1888 and editor of *The Veterinary Record*, died in October 1913 aged sixty-seven. He has a special place in this history as one of a small number of Victorian veterinary surgeons who, by example and unceasing endeavour, created a competent profession that had pride and high ideals. Everybody loved him, for they knew that he was fearless, fair, kind and true. His gift for communication by word or pen enabled him constantly to help his colleagues in their search for professional identity. His influence for good was incalculable, for, week by week, *The Veterinary Record* brought news and comment to every veterinary surgeon in the kingdom. There could be no finer tribute than the respect and affection he inspired in students, as their examiner; always, he encouraged them to recall that trifle he knew they knew but had momentarily overlooked. In 1907 the profession presented him with the portrait that graces RCVS Headquarters in Belgrave Square. He was a kindly, gentle man, but too generous to have a big balance at the bank. When he died, close friends petitioned for a Civil List pension for his children. This was granted in 1915 (the first to dependants of a veterinary surgeon): "Miss Louisa Hunting, Mr Frederick Charles Hunting (jointly and to the survivor of them) in consideration of the services rendered to veterinary science by their father, the late Mr William Hunting F.R.C.V.S., and of their inadequate means of support, £50."

The future of *The Veterinary Record* was secured after William Hunting's death through the generosity of W.H. Brown, proprietor of H. & W. Brown, who had printed and published every issue. A remarkable rapport developed between Hunting and Brown, to the extent that Brown was not only business manager, but also sub-editor, and occasionally contributed abstracts and translations from French journals. When Hunting died, Brown purchased the goodwill of the journal, and continued its publication until 1920, when, through his efforts, it was transferred to the National Veterinary Medical Association. Brown's admiration for Hunting is explicit in a note in *The Record* for 8th November 1913, shortly after Hunting's death: "Those who have worked with him are continuing the work, and his known views on most professional matters will be followed so far as they are not affected by changing conditions of professional work . . . in all respects *The Record* will continue as heretofore 'A weekly journal for the profession.' "

*   *   *

The story of veterinary involvement in the First World War is told in the 'Official History of the War, Royal Army Veterinary Services.' From 1914 to 1918 some 3,200,000 horses, mules, bullocks and camels were in the veterinary care of some 1,300 officers and 42,000 other ranks. As in every calling at that time, men and women gave and gave to protect their country. The RCVS was continuously in consultation with the War Office, and several high-ranking veterinary officers served on the Council. On the Home Front practitioners helped each other through local veterinary associations, so that the younger could serve with the Forces while the older looked after practices for their neighbours.

At a basic level, the physical labour of veterinary practice was recognised in a letter dated 12th April 1918, from J.S. Leaver of the Supplementary Ration Section of the Ministry of Food, to the Secretary of the RCVS: "Veterinary Surgeons are included in the list of those persons entitled to the Supplementary Ration. They are graded under class 'D'."

At a lofty level, on 29th November 1918 Major-General L.J. Blenkinsop, Director-General of the Army Veterinary Services, relayed from the War Office to all veterinary personnel a message from General Sir John S. Cowans: "On the occasion of His Majesty the King being graciously pleased to raise the Army Veterinary Corps to the status of a 'Royal' Corps, the Quartermaster-General of the Forces wishes to convey to all ranks his congratulations and appreciation of the good work they have performed during the present war."

Remembrance is warming — irrespective of the level of recall.

CHAPTER 16

Veterinary research in 1922 — The first veterinary lady.

Three historically important matters reached maturity within four years of the 1918 Armistice. Each had beginnings in the 19th century, and maturation of each was influenced by the war.

One was recognition of the urgent need for veterinary research, implicit in the Report of 1922 by the Advisory Committee on Research into Diseases in Animals. A second was entry of the first woman into the British veterinary profession, in December 1922. The third was the birth in 1919 of the National Veterinary Medical Association, a professional organisation to operate beyond the restricted terms of reference (competence and probity) of the RCVS.

First, veterinary research.

If research is defined as systematic investigation of observed phenomena, there was no veterinary research in Britain before the 1860's. Early volumes of *The Veterinarian* published many clinical papers, but it was unusual for more than one case to be described and rare for the picture to be amplified by post mortem examination. The closest approach to research was investigation of farm animal diseases by James Beart Simonds, Professor of Cattle Pathology at the London veterinary school, on behalf of the Royal Agricultural Society of England.

The cattle plague epidemic of 1865/66 was an agricultural and financial catastrophe but it had two redeeming veterinary consequences. First, it stressed the special problem of controlling animal plagues by emphasising the difference between medical and veterinary handling of infectious diseases: in human medicine, treatment is essential to save life, while in the veterinary field infection is eliminated by isolation and slaughter. Secondly, it made veterinary surgeons *think* about a specific disease. What was the cause of cattle plague? Where had it come from? How did it spread? To pose a question is the first step in research, to seek an answer is the second, and it was now manifest that research was

147

essential to avoid similar calamities in the future. Coincidentally, Pasteur was developing techniques for probing biological problems, and the tools of the laboratory — the microscope, measuring instruments, glassware, chemicals, and the like — were coming within common reach.

An episode of this period with marginal relevance to veterinary research, was the establishment in the Wandsworth Road, London, in July 1871, of the Brown Institution. Thomas Brown, M.A., LL.B., citizen of London and Dublin, died in 1852, bequeathing to the University of London £20,000 to found "an Animal Sanatory Institution situated within a mile of Westminster or Southwark." The Institution was to be concerned with "investigating, studying, and without charge beyond immediate expenses, endeavouring to cure maladies, distempers, and injuries, any Quadripeds or Birds useful to man may be found subject to." Dr J. Burdon-Sanderson was the first Professor-Superintendent, with William Duguid, MRCVS, his veterinary assistant.

The Institution was chronically short of money and equipment, and has well-nigh been forgotten, although a number of men who used its laboratories for longer or shorter periods over half-a-century, made significant contributions to medical knowledge (notably Victor Horsley and Charles Sherrington during the decade from 1884). Although Brown's intention was investigation of animal diseases, this was broadly interpreted by a succession of medical Superintendents and medical bias left veterinary people in the animal clinic rather than the laboratory. It is of veterinary interest, however, that readers of the first volume of *The Veterinary Journal* in 1875 were invited to send specimens to the Brown Institution for examination and report.

True veterinary research in Britain began with John McFadyean — already introduced into this history — who was undisputed leader of the profession for thirty years from his appointment as principal of the London school in 1894. McFadyean's veterinary, medical and scientific training to 1883 has been described, as also has his establishment of a course in pathology and bacteriology at the Edinburgh veterinary school, and his founding in 1888 of *The Journal of Comparative Pathology and Therapeutics*. It may be noted that McFadyean was the only veterinary surgeon in Britain equipped to take immediate advantage of the great biological discoveries made in Europe during the last two decades of the nineteenth century. It is emphasised, too, that his exceptional gifts were unrelated to his medical training. McFadyean was first and always a veterinary surgeon; he pursued the medical course in Edinburgh to acquire instruction in pathology and bacteriology, that was not available at any British veterinary school. He was not interested in human medicine or surgery, and could be cuttingly caustic about what he considered the shortcomings of the medical profession.

As Principal of the London school, McFadyean had the absolute confidence of its Governors. It might have been supposed, therefore, that they would have ensured that his researches were based on a good laboratory and adequate assistance.

No supposition could be wider of the mark.

McFadyean's over-crowded laboratory was continuously on the verge of starvation. Equipment had to be used, and used, and used again. Cash was counted in shillings. Rabies, anthrax, tuberculosis, glanders and other dangerous diseases were dealt with in wholly inadequate conditions, and only McFadyean's rigid rules for laboratory safety prevented infection of the staff. This poverty of the research laboratory reflected the penury of the whole school that was still, in the early twentieth century, dependent on students' fees for survival. There was a small income from manufacture of tuberculin and mallein (the diagnostic agents of tuberculosis and glanders, respectively) and from the school's practice, and a life-saving annual grant from the Royal Agricultural Society, but no Governmental support whatever — in contrast to generously State-aided veterinary schools across the Channel.

It is a historical enigma, that decade after decade, the Governors of the London veterinary school — among them, always, great landowners and wealthy men, all presumably interested in the progress of veterinary science — would annually approve the work of the school and ignore the bread-line budget. Their responsibility seemed to end at the Board-room door.

If no account be taken of an insanitary room below street level in Old Scotland Yard, where, at the turn of the century, pig entrails were examined for evidence of swine fever, it can be said that the first support by Government for veterinary research was in 1905. Stewart Stockman had recently been appointed Chief Veterinary Officer (on McFadyean's recommendation), and had persuaded Mr Ailwyn Fellowes, President of the Board of Agriculture and Fisheries, to create a committee with McFadyean as Chairman, to investigate contagious abortion in cattle. Little was known about this disease, except that it was produced by a micro-organism, but in many parts of the country it was the cause of abortion of calves and consequent loss of the milk that their dams should have produced. A modest Treasury grant covered rent of a house called 'The Poplars' at Sudbury in Middlesex, three rooms of which were converted into the first Government veterinary laboratory. The research progressed to an extent that warranted expansion in 1908 into the more ample premises of Alperton Lodge, Alperton, also in Middlesex. This house had outbuildings, stables and eight acres of land. The researches on contagious abortion, actively led by McFadyean and Stockman, continued to prosper, and investigations began on other diseases. By 1911 the value of veterinary research was officially recognised, but cash investment was still small.

Government money for development of the British economy was released by the Development and Road Fund Improvement Act of 1909, under which a Development Commission was established in May 1910, with help to agriculture heading its priority list. McFadyean tapped this source for the first-ever Government grant to the London veterinary school. The sum involved was £1,390, for studies on bovine tuberculosis (£650), scrapie disease of sheep (£230), Johne's disease of cattle (£410), and toxicity of the salts of zinc (£100). Through the same fund, Stockman was granted £28,000 in 1914 to build "a well-equipped and up-to-date laboratory . . . in a convenient position outside London," with £2,000 annually for maintenance.

Stockman's chosen site was of forty acres at New Haw, Weybridge in Surrey. Building began in 1914, but war-time difficulties delayed completion until 1917. On 25th September of that year, with "the premises . . . scarcely out of the hands of the contractors," Stockman (who had been knighted in 1913) acted as host to the Midland Counties, Royal Counties, and Central Veterinary Medical Associations. "Sir Stewart personally conducted the party round and explained some of the important work." The visitors were enormously impressed. The excitement is unmistakable in *The Veterinary Record's* report of that day, for at Weybridge, for the first time in Britain, practising veterinary surgeons could actually see, instead of visualising, the scientific development of their profession. In his vote of thanks, John Malcolm, President of the Midland Counties Association, referred to "the finest buildings of the kind in the world."

A consequence of the urge to survive in war, is recognition of life's true necessities. The First World War taught Britain sharply that she could be blockaded and starved. More food must be home-produced — more milk, more meat, more grain. Veterinary science was an essential part of animal production, and Governmental support for veterinary research was continued, and extended, when the war was over.

The Advisory Committee on Research into Diseases in Animals, was appointed by the Development Commission in November 1920. Eight members, including McFadyean, were under the chairmanship of Sir David Prain, with the terms of reference: "To report on the facilities now available for the scientific study of the diseases of animals, to indicate what extension of those facilities is desirable in the immediate future . . . and to advise as to the steps which should be taken to secure the aid of competent scientific workers in investigating diseases in animals." The Committee met fifteen times and received evidence from twenty-four individuals, before issuing in 1922 a Report that opened many eyes.

The estimated value of cattle, sheep and pigs in the United Kingdom in 1920 was £400,000,000. The estimated annual loss from disease was £5,000,000. The amount of State subsidy in 1920–21 for research at the five veterinary schools (London, Liverpool, Edinburgh, Glasgow, Dublin) was £3,696. The Committee's comment was that "such a condition of affairs constitutes a national disgrace." For 1921–22, £128,000 had been earmarked for agricultural research, £39,600 for fishery research, and £9,000 for veterinary research (essentially at the Weybridge laboratories). There were only five full-time veterinary research workers in the United Kingdom, three in McFadyean's laboratory, and two at Weybridge. All other veterinary research was on a part-time basis.

The Committee believed "that an essential part of any scheme for the improvement of veterinary research is the gradual creation, with varying assistance from State funds, of a cadre of research workers with those definite prospects of tenure, pay, promotion and superannuation benefits essential to ensure their recruitment." This was the first official admission that veterinary scientists must eat.

For the London school, the Committee recommended "construction of new laboratories at the earliest possible date." This was given priority over a proposal to establish a Research Institute in Comparative Pathology at Cambridge. The Cambridge scheme would be justified, they considered, "should financial conditions become easier."

They welcomed the creation by private subscription of the Animal Diseases Research Association in Scotland, and its support by the Development Commission in the form of "two teams of workers based on the Veterinary Colleges at Edinburgh and Glasgow during the first year." They advised that "whatever the fate of this particular scheme, permanent facilities should be provided in Scotland commensurate with the problems awaiting study and the economic issues at stake."

Finally, and at some length, they recommended (McFadyean dissenting) appointment of a "Diseases of Animals Research Committee (or Board)" to advise on "all applications for advances from the Development Fund." In an Appendix to the Report, McFadyean explained that he was opposed to an advisory committee because it would be "not unlike the creation of a general staff almost equal in numbers to the rest of an army." Unsaid, was that he believed passionately that a competent research worker is the best judge of his own problem, and that committee advice is less likely to help than to irritate.

No sooner had this Report been published, than it became known that a large sum of money, the Corn Repeal Fund created by the Corn Production Act (Repeal) Act of 1921, had become available for agricultural (including veterinary) research. Financial constraints on the Prain Committee's recommendations vanished. £32,000 was made available for a Pathological Research Institute at the London school, and a slightly larger sum for a similar Institute in Cambridge. A Cambridge Professorship in Animal Pathology was endowed with another £30,000. There was a special grant for research on foot-and-mouth disease. Veterinary Advisers were appointed to Cardiff, Bangor, and Newcastle-upon-Tyne, and two veterinary research scholarships annually, each tenable for three years, invited young men to embrace veterinary research as a lifetime's career.

Within months, McFadyean's shoestring was of a bygone age.

*   *   *

So much for research. Enter now the ladies.

The Veterinary Journal of 1889 reported that "a clever and learned Parisienne" who "went through a course of veterinary surgery and medicine," was not expected to treat horses, but to follow "the lighter labour of alleviating the sufferings of sick lap-dogs." In the same year, "Fräulein Stephanie Kruszewska, a Polish lady . . . graduated with distinction at Zurich Veterinary Institute," and in 1894 a correspondent to *The Veterinary Record* (signing himself 'Dystokia'), noted a proposal to found a veterinary college for women in America, and commented: "Ladies might do very well in some directions, but I ask myself how about rough country practice?"

These reports summarise the attitude of veterinary surgeons of the nineteenth century to the prospect of female colleagues. The barrier was physical, not intellectual. It was irrelevant to refer to attempts by women to enter the medical profession, because in human medicine women — as women — had special talents. They did not have special skills for the "rough country practice" that was by far the greatest part of the veterinary world. Indeed, apart from the occasional Amazon, the physical strength required, say, to castrate half-a-dozen fractious colts, or to turn in the womb a breech-presenting calf, was beyond them. It is fairy-tale to represent the ladies of those days as Joans of Arc seeking veterinary justice for their sex. Female veterinary surgeons only became relevant when there were opportunities to specialise in small animal practice, teaching, research, and preventive veterinary medicine.

In October 1895 Principal William Williams of the New veterinary school in Edinburgh, accepted Aleen Isabel Cust as a pupil, the first female veterinary student in the United Kingdom. She worked diligently, and in due course applied to sit the RCVS professional examination at the end of the first year. Her application was refused by the RCVS, because it was "contrary to long usage and all precedent that women should be admitted to the veterinary profession."

Aleen Cust was disappointed, but continued her studies.

Meanwhile, Principal Williams and his son Professor William Owen Williams, decided to test the validity in law of the stand taken by the RCVS. The case came before Lord Kincairney in Edinburgh in the latter half of 1897. As a preliminary, the RCVS pleaded that that court had no jurisdiction over a corporate body without property in Scotland, and domiciled in London. RCVS counsel went on to argue that there was no objection to Principal Williams admitting whom he liked to his school, but the RCVS was not bound, indeed not entitled, to give its diploma to ladies. The objective of the action was to obtain an answer to the latter part of the argument, but the plea of no jurisdiction had first to be considered. In the event, after much cogitation and close examination of all relevant material, Lord Kincairney "sustained the plea of no jurisdiction, with some little regret, because when the action had been brought it might have been decided here as well as in London . . . As he had, in his opinion, no jurisdiction, it would not be fitting that he should express any opinion about the pursuers' title, still less about the interesting question on its merits."

Aleen Cust completed the course at Williams's school, but left without the RCVS diploma. It would be exaggeration to say that the RCVS was delighted by the 'no jurisdiction' ending to the Aleen Cust case, but they did not view it with disfavour. At that time, veterinary ladies seemed irrelevant.

During the next two decades the RCVS received, and politely sidestepped, occasional requests for information as to how ladies might enter the profession (notably from Liverpool University in 1915). Fall of the citadel was by action beyond control — the reward of a grateful Government to all women for valour and endurance in the First World War. At the RCVS meeting on 9th January 1920, Secretary Bullock reported that the Sex Disqualification (Removal) Act had been passed by Parliament. Aleen Cust applied to sit the final examination, supported "by testimonials and recommendations from members of the profession." In

December 1922 she became the first female British veterinary surgeon. She is affectionately remembered by a research scholarship that bears her name.

*   *   *

Before considering the foundation of the National Veterinary Medical Association (the third of three important veterinary advances stimulated by the First World War), homage must be paid to Frank Walls Garnett who died in August 1922. Frank Garnett was a great RCVS President, yet is indistinctly recalled because his work was untouched by personal or professional publicity. He was first elected to the RCVS Council in 1904, became particularly involved with Parliamentary business, and was closely associated with McFadyean in the long struggle for a statutory registration fee, embodied in the Veterinary Surgeons' Act (1881) Amendment Act of 1920. He was President of the RCVS for five consecutive years throughout the First World War, rarely missed a Council or Committee meeting, in spite of living in Windermere, and maintained the highest standards of chairmanship. He wrote "Westmorland Agriculture 1800 – 1900," a splendidly illustrated and authoritative study of the people who lived around his home.

*   *   *

It has been briefly noted that the roots of the National Veterinary Medical Association (NVMA), were in the territorial veterinary associations, the first of which was founded in 1851. An important step towards the NVMA was formation of the National Veterinary Association (NVA) at the time of the British National Veterinary Congress of 1881. There was no link between the NVA and the local associations. The NVA was simply a non-territorial association, to which any veterinary surgeon might belong on payment of half-a-guinea, that met "in different parts of the kingdom, from time to time . . . under the management of a local 'Provisional Committee.' "

As the years passed it became increasingly clear that a professional association was needed to deal with matters outside the terms of reference of the RCVS. William Hunting was among the first to realise, in 1892, that "in the National Veterinary Association might be found the nucleus of a really national body." He drew attention to "the value to the medical practitioner of that great organization The British Medical Association," and declared: "We have to influence public opinion, we have to advance our corporate interests, we have to show a reason for our existence, and all this is more easily done by association than by individual effort."

William Hunting, and others, found, however, that national organisation of some three thousand individualistic veterinary gentlemen, many with strong ties to local associations, was more readily said than achieved.

The prospect of a national professional association came, and went, and came again. Years passed. Finally, on 27th January 1909 Professor Orlando Charnock Bradley, of the Edinburgh veterinary school, put to the Scottish Metropolitan Veterinary Medical Society proposals for "formation of one single British Veterinary Association," based on the suggestion that existing territorial societies should become Divisions affiliated to the National Association. Bradley declared that: "The National Association forms a very substantial foundation for a British Veterinary Association." Formally, he moved: "That this Society is in favour of the principle of amalgamation of Veterinary Societies, and that a circular letter be sent to the Veterinary Societies in the United Kingdom asking for expression of their views."

The Veterinary Record enthusiastically supported Bradley's "radical and attractive" proposals, and emphasised what everyone knew, but some found hard to admit, that: "A successful amalgamation of all our societies under the 'National' would . . . be of incalculable benefit to the whole profession."

Reaction from the local societies was, in general, favourable, but progress towards union could not be described as impetuous. By August 1913 *The Veterinary Record* noted that the NVA was acting "through its Council" as the "centre of the organisation of the Societies," but no more had been achieved a year later when war was declared.

As happens in war, the present is so distasteful that minds turn to the future: at all costs, it must be better than the past. So with the amalgamation of veterinary societies. Everyone was ready for the meeting of 31st October 1919 that accepted the principle of a National Veterinary Medical Association, "drafted deliberately upon the lines of the British Medical Association." *The Veterinary Record* said of that meeting: "Optimism was the prevailing note."

The NVMA took over *The Veterinary Record* from W.H. Brown, who had scrupulously maintained its principles and format since William Hunting's death. A new era for that journal began with a message from Charnock Bradley, first President of the NVMA, of which the reference is:-

"1st January 1921: New Series: Volume I, Number 1, Page 1."

CHAPTER 17

Veterinary schools overseas — The RCVS library

There was no renunciation of the past in the NVMA's 'New Series' *Veterinary Record* of 1921, only anticipation of the future. It was symbolic, however, of a new era separated by war from another world, hopefully better, certainly different.

So with the RCVS. A new maturity of that body is detectable at this time, reflecting not only the common stimulus of having "won the war," but also the novel security of an assured income through the statutory annual registration fee vouchsafed by the Veterinary Surgeons' Act (1881) Amendment Act of 1920.

In June 1920, however, a few months before the Amendment Bill had achieved Parliamentary approval, the RCVS was attacked by *The Times* newspaper for alleged failure to provide adequate veterinary education. The inspiration for this criticism is obscure, but its impact was trebled by a follow-up letter from J. George Adami, Vice-Chancellor of Liverpool University. Adami, born in Lancashire in 1862 of distant Italian stock, had been professor of Pathology at McGill University in Canada from 1892 until twelve months previously. His letter of 12th June 1920 to *The Times* said: "I am grateful to you for taking up this matter of university degrees for veterinary surgeons and the improvement of the status of the veterinary profession. What obstructions stand in the way of our universities in their endeavours to develop higher courses in veterinary medicine cannot be realized by Parliament and the general public. These obstructions are due to the . . . inertia of the Royal College of Veterinary Surgeons. It is intolerable that courses of instruction rendering a candidate eligible to practise as a veterinary surgeon can only be given by the universities of this country provided they receive the approval of the Royal College of Veterinary Surgeons. In order to establish a school of veterinary science, this University, in 1904, was compelled to buy out a Scottish proprietary school with its sign manual . . ." and ". . . was placed in the humiliating position of having to appoint on to its staff the proprietor of the sign manual, wholly irrespective of his academic qualifications . . . These facts . . . justify . . . a searching inquiry into the state of veterinary science in Great Britain and the extent to which it is served by the Royal College."

It would be improper to describe the statements of a university Vice-Chancellor as scurrilous, but it can fairly be said that Adami's point of view might have been more diplomatically expressed. His explanation of the manner of acquisition by Liverpool University of William Owen Williams's sign manual in 1904, is of historical interest because it confirms what the RCVS suspected and the University denied at the time, that the long-term objective was to establish not only a teaching but also a licensing veterinary school in Liverpool. There is regrettable injustice in Adami's inference that William Owen Williams (long since deceased) did not match up to university standards, for it will be recalled that it was Williams's interest in veterinary education that achieved the first specialist veterinary qualification, the Diploma in Veterinary State Medicine.

Reply to *The Times* and J. George Adami came from John McFadyean, who deferred to no one and cared only for the truth. He turned on Adami, via *The Times*, in frigid fury. The exchange of letters left outsiders bewildered. Charge and counter-charge. Why? No obvious reason has been found, because veterinary men of the day were as competent as graduates in other callings. Further, in London, Edinburgh and Liverpool veterinary students could opt to take a concurrent university degree to add to the MRCVS diploma. So why this sudden accusation of incompetence? It would seem that in the post-war scramble for money and facilities, envious eyes were cast on veterinary students still outside the university system. Envy, rationalised as proselytism, was expressed, Adami-fashion, in doctored indignation and the need for "searching inquiry into the state of veterinary science in Great Britain."

The envious eyes belonged to powerful and persistent people.

Shortly after this episode, but in unrelated business, the RCVS Council considered the desirability of allowing teachers to act as internal examiners (forbidden by the 1844 Charter), and of being permitted to appoint as examiners veterinary surgeons who did not possess the Fellowship diploma (forbidden by the 1876 Charter). After discussion, a Draft Supplementary Charter to cover these two simple modifications in the examination rules was submitted to the Privy Council. To the amazement of the RCVS, London and Liverpool Universities lodged protests, not against the terms of the proposed Charter, but against what London called "the monopoly of the Royal College" to grant a licence to practise veterinary medicine and surgery. RCVS Councillors were further startled by a letter dated 23rd November 1921 from Almeric Fitzroy of the Privy Council Office, warning that the RCVS "would be well advised if they came into line with the policy advocated by the Universities . . . as otherwise the only alternative may prove to be . . . a searching enquiry . . . which might easily lead to great changes in the powers and privileges of the College."

The treasured "one portal" of entry into the profession, vital gateway to universal competence, triumph of the 1881 Act, was under siege, Nationwide resistance within the profession was epitomized by Principal Charnock Bradley (M.D., D.Sc., F.R.C.V.S.) of the Edinburgh veterinary school, in an address to the NVMA's Scottish Metropolitan Division on 25th October 1922: "During the past 78 years the body politic and corporate has conscientiously guarded the public interest to the utmost limit of its powers . . . the . . . one portal and one portal only . . . of all imaginable modes of entry . . . is the best, as ensuring uniformity of standard by which the public may assess the qualifications of candidates for their favour."

The RCVS briefed Counsel to advise on their reply to Almeric Fitzroy of the Privy Council Office. Their case was "heard by a Committee of the Privy Council," and in a communication dated 24th July 1922 they were informed that "modification of the terms of the Draft Supplementary Charter in the way proposed by the University of London and the University of Liverpool was *ultra vires*, and could only be effected by legislation." It was stated, further, that "consideration of the Draft Supplemental Charter . . . will now be proceeded with."

The Charter was granted without further fuss in 1923, but the "one portal" had been preserved by technicality, not by change of heart; it was reprieve, not victory.

*   *   *

The Veterinary Surgeons' Act (1881) provided for registration with the RCVS of colonial and foreign veterinary surgeons holding recognised diplomas, subject to approval by the RCVS and the Privy Council. No action was taken for several years, however, and the first occasion on which such registration was considered appears to have been at a meeting of the RCVS Council on 12th October 1887. The Secretary read a letter "from a graduate of Columbia Veterinary College, asking whether the diplomas of that College were recognised" by the RCVS. Councillor Walley of the Edinburgh school "said he had had applications from various colleges in America and Canada, and he thought it was high time that it should be determined what colleges were to be recognised." However, a committee created to consider the matter failed to meet, and fifteen months later President Pritchard "thought it had been allowed to lapse." It was then formally resurrected to consider an application from J.H. Steel, MRCVS, for recognition of his veterinary school in Bombay; it reported some five months later, Applications for recognition from Ontario and Victoria had been considered in addition to that from Bombay, but as there had been "no guide whatever as to the period of study . . . nor . . . any indication of the nature and extent of the education" it was "impossible . . . for the committee to take any . . . steps." The Secretary was instructed "to write to the various colonial and foreign schools with a view of obtaining prospectuses." This had been done, prospectuses had been examined, and, for the first time, the position of graduates from veterinary schools outside the United Kingdom had been closely examined — and an embarrassing discovery had to be reported to the RCVS Council on 9th January 1890.

The Committee had found that no British school had correctly interpreted RCVS Bye-law 35, based on the 1881 Act: "A student holding a foreign or colonial veterinary diploma from any veterinary examining body recognised by the Council, should be exempt from attendance on the course of lectures for the first two years, and from the examinations at the end of those years respectively." The words "recognised by the Council" had been overlooked. The MRCVS course at that time was of three years, and all the schools had been granting two years' exemption to every graduate from any colonial or foreign veterinary school, not one of which had been formally recognised by the RCVS. As President Axe regretted: "We have evidently been going astray . . . the College has been erring in examining such students."

In further discussion it transpired that not many men from overseas had thus acquired the MRCVS diploma, but Councillor Brown was concerned for "two gentlemen" at the London school "with Canadian diplomas, who paid their fees on the clear understanding that they would be examined at the end of the sessional course, as they knew that other persons similarly situated had been examined previously." Finally, Councillor McCall's pragmatic suggestion was accepted that, in future, schools should refuse exemption of study to veterinary graduates of unrecognised schools, but that, as an act of grace, "students now at the schools" should "be examined in the usual way." It was agreed, however, that the credentials of all colonial and foreign schools must now be scrutinised, and that "students would only be admitted from schools whose curriculum is equal . . . to our own."

This principle was followed thereafter. It was tested in 1896 by a request from the Melbourne veterinary school for full recognition "when equality of teaching and examination etc. had been established . . . graduates of the the Melbourne Veterinary College . . . to practise in any part of the British Empire the same as . . . members of the Royal College of Veterinary Surgeons." An RCVS committee elected to adjudicate on this request, reported on 13th January 1897 that "the standard generally was not up to that of the Royal College," and advised against an undertaking about future recognition, because "views might differ as to whether the terms of any such bargain could be complied with."

Further applications for recognition by the Melbourne veterinary school (backed by the Government of Victoria), were refused in 1898, 1902, 1909, 1910, 1911 and 1916, all on the grounds that the training in Melbourne was inferior to that in Britain. *The Veterinary Record* followed these episodes closely, and supported the action taken by the RCVS up to the time of the application of 28th June 1916, prepared by Dean Harold Woodruff. After the Council meeting of 6th October 1916, at which that application was considered, the *Record* doubted RCVS impartiality, and considered that the reasons for refusing the application were "anything but convincing." It was added, however, that the memorial from Melbourne contained "apparent reticence on some important points."

The Australians, highly dissatisfied, referred to the Privy Council, as a test case, the application to the RCVS of H.R. Seddon, Esq., B.V.Sc., Melbourne, for registration as a Colonial Practitioner. To their dismay, early in 1917, Seddon's appeal was dismissed.

The Melbourne/RCVS story was not unique, but has been given in some detail because it exemplifies the inflexible stand taken by the RCVS against recognition of any school at which the training was considered inferior to its own. In retrospect, its action seems a mite stuffy, but the intention was sound, and certainly provided world-wide notice that the RCVS diploma would not be granted lightly.

As with so many matters, war hastened solution of this nagging problem. After the Armistice, the RCVS agreed, as an emergency measure, to give to ex-service colonial veterinary graduates from any school exemption from three years of the four-year MRCVS course. A considerable number of men took advantage of this gesture of goodwill, and the foundation was laid for further negotiation. In July 1922 the RCVS referred to a special committee "the general question of the conditions under which foreign and colonial Veterinary Degrees and Diplomas should be recognised . . . with instructions to report as soon as possible." On the advice of this committee, the Council decided in April 1923 to institute "reciprocal arrangements . . . with regard to recognition of Colonial Diplomas." These, in essence, were that colonial four-year-course graduates would receive the RCVS diploma after one year at a British school, and that MsRCVS would receive a colonial diploma after one year at a four-year-course colonial school.

Discussion of the more complex problem of establishing criteria for recognising foreign (as distinct from colonial) veterinary schools, appears to have been avoided by successive RCVS Councils down the years. Indeed, in reply to a letter of 14th November 1928 from the Privy Council, seeking clarification on "reciprocal recognition of veterinary qualifications, in a proposed International Convention on the treatment of foreigners," Secretary Bullock could provide only the standard reference to Section 13 of the 1881 Veterinary Surgeons' Act. He assured their Lordships, however, that the RCVS "would be prepared to recognise . . . any veterinary diploma . . . awarded after a course of training . . . not inferior to the course . . . required of British subjects in this country." The good Secretary prayed, no doubt, that Solomon would be at hand to advise on so invidious a decision.

*   *   *

Chief Veterinary Officer Stewart Stockman died suddenly in 1926 aged fifty-seven. Thus ended two decades of benevolent domination, with his father-in-law John McFadyean, of the British veterinary profession. It was the profession's good fortune that both were men of integrity, for they shared the highest positions in veterinary education, research, and Governmental and professional administration from 1905 to 1926. Stockman's outstanding contribution was development of a Government veterinary field and laboratory service second to none in the world, reflecting scientific and administrative acumen, and the trust of Government. During his leadership there were some sixty-one Acts and Orders of veterinary relevance, many initiated by him, or, through him, by McFadyean. In 1910 he joined McFadyean as co-editor of *The Journal of Comparative Pathology and Therapeutics*, in which they published, separately or jointly, some sixty-five scientific papers, many being definitive descriptions of important diseases. Their researches covered glanders, Johne's disease, tuberculosis, anthrax, epizootic abortion (especially development of the diagnostic agglutination test), foot-and-mouth disease, scrapie, parasitic pneumonia, louping-ill, pregnancy toxaemia, joint-ill, piroplasmosis, botriomycosis, abortion in mares, sheep scab, tumours, and ragwort poisoning. They discovered the disease-producing organisms *Vibrio fetus* and *Babesia divergens*.

McFadyean's dismay at the loss of his son-in-law is revealed in the opening words of the obituary in his *Journal*: "It is with infinite regret that we record the death of Sir Stewart Stockman . . ." It was, indeed, an irreparable loss, and influenced his decision to retire from the Principalship of the London school twelve months later. His ambition to have a fine research laboratory had been realised in 1925, when the new Institute of Pathology attached to the school was opened on 14th July by the Duke of Connaught. Collaboration through Stockman with the Ministry's laboratories at Weybridge had been part of the plan for development of the Institute, but it was now a reminder of what might have been, rather than a challenge for the future.

*   *   *

At the end of the Council meeting on 4th July 1919, a proposal by Councillor Garnett was accepted unanimously that a special committee should "consider the question of a Memorial to those of our Profession who have fallen in the War." This committee established a War Memorial Fund, first to purchase a "simple and inexpensive" memorial tablet recording the names of those who had died on active service, and secondly (using the bulk of the Fund) to improve, extend and endow the library at RCVS head-quarters, "to be designated The War Memorial Library, with a reading room accessible at all times to the members of the profession."

Provision of an adequate library had been a elusive objective since acquisition of the first permanent home for the RCVS at No. 10 Red Lion Square in 1853. At a Council meeting on 14th December of that year, the House Committee were "happy to state that . . . on the first floor are four rooms well calculated for Council and Board rooms, Library and Museum," and within a month considerable donations of books and specimens had been received.

In its early years, however, the RCVS library suffered the fate of inanimate objects left to their own devices: it fell into disarray, was half-heartedly pulled together, slipped back into confusion. For years no record was kept of books, reports and pamphlets received. A Hunting editorial in *The Veterinary Record* of 20th September 1890 declared that the library "wants thoroughly overhauling. It contains many books of value together with not a little rubbish . . . no printed catalogue exists, no arrangement of works on the shelves is attempted, and as to any classification of the books — such . . . has never been thought of." Some eighteen months later, the Library and Museum Committee proposed purchase of two book-cases, and Councillor Raymond hoped this would be approved "because the appearance of the place . . . is something very dreadful."

In 1894 Secretary Hill was appointed Librarian. The library was to be open from ten in the morning until four in the afternoon, unless required for Council meetings. Loans were not permitted, so that use of the library was restricted, virtually, to veterinary surgeons in London. Little happened to alleviate this literary anaemia until the magificent trans-fusion in 1900 of George Fleming's professional library. In his letter of 10th March of that year making the offer to the RCVS, Fleming wrote: "I am not quite certain how many volumes the library contains, but I think there are not less than 600. The books are in several languages and many of them are very rare and have been the collection of a lifetime." It is a measure of minimal interest in the library, coupled with RCVS indigence at the time, that this splendid collection was not catalogued until 1904, and that binding of presented journals was not even discussed (let alone agreed) until 1906. At a meeting of the Central Veterinary Medical Association in June 1907, McFadyean described the RCVS library as "utterly unworthy of the name," and that of the London school as "no better."

The appointment of Fred Bullock as RCVS Secretary on 1st February 1907, placed the library in the care of a scholar. He was twenty-nine, educated at Stafford Grammar School and the Université de Caen. He had been for ten years Chief Clerk in charge of the Staffordshire Higher Education Department, and for seven years County Council Inspector of Commercial Evening Schools. He taught French in the Stafford County Technical School, and had founded the Cercle Français de Stafford. Frenchmen described his command of their language as "marvellous." He had a special interest in history. Clearly, the library would prosper in such hands. The title of 'Librarian' lapsed when Secretary Hill retired, and Bullock was not thus designated until October 1919. He was librarian in all but name, however, from the day he joined the RCVS, and his influence within a few months of appointment is detectable in an urgent search for a scheme to permit the less precious of the library's estimated 2,000 books to be available on loan. With regret, however, it was decided that this was impossible until there was money to recruit a "proper librarian."

Only lack of funds now restricted development of a worthwhile profes-sional library. Bullock's interest stimulated presentations in ever-increasing volume, and borrowing schemes were discussed on many occasions, but the recurrent conclusion was that voiced by McFadyean in

1913: "We should have to appoint a librarian to do that, and we cannot afford it." *The Veterinary Record* of 31st October 1914 drew attention to an advertisement prepared by Bullock asking, on behalf of the library, for "gifts of certain specified publications, chiefly journals, which are needed to complete series." Earlier neglect is emphasised by inclusion in this list of "several volumes of our one English journal of comparative pathology;" this was, of course, McFadyean's *Journal* founded in 1888, of which he had conscientiously given copies to the library, some of which must have gone astray. Publication of this list is proof that by this time Bullock had personally examined the entire contents of the library.

Bullock's first Report as official Librarian was for the the year ending 31st March 1922, and was presented to the RCVS Annual General Meeting in June of that year. President Bradley described it as "marking an epoch," and added: "It shows the great progress made towards the establishment of a central library for the profession." The Report reflects Bullock's enthusiasm, in spite of shortage of money, bookcases and furniture. The number of readers during the year had been "about 50." Some ninety books and periodicals had been borrowed under a lending scheme agreed in July 1921. It was hoped that "the general office staff will be sufficient to cope with the daily routine' of the library.

The opening of the War Memorial Library by the Right Honourable L.C.M.S Amery on 7th June 1928, was a considerable occasion. The necessary funds had been subscribed by the profession, together with a grant in aid from the Carnegie Trust. As Secretary of State for Dominion Affairs and the Colonies, Mr Amery "enthusiastically welcomed the establishing of the War Memorial Library, an instrument for scientific work, the foremost in the British Empire." *The Veterinary Record* expressed the profession's pride not only in the library itself, but also in "the spirit in which it was conceived and created," expressed in "the motto 'Pro Patria, 1914–1918' which adorns the mantelpiece."

*   *   *

As will have been realised, the RCVS had little thought for luxuries in a struggle for survival of three-score-and-sixteen years. Access in 1920 to an assured, if modest, income caused change in bank balance and professional confidence. Councillor Bradley's proposition of January 1926 was greeted, therefore, with enthusiasm: "That it be remitted to the Chairmen's Committee to consider the question of the adoption of academic dress for Fellows and Members of the College."

Over the years, through the generosity of individuals, the RCVS Council had acquired some of the outward signs of collective dignity. A

Presidential Chair from Councillor Greaves in 1887; a Mace from President Williams, and a Presidential Robe from the whole Council, in 1903; a Chain of Office from Councillor Dollar in 1904. Academic dress for the entire profession was a much more ambitious matter, but promulgated with alacrity. The Chairmen's Committee to which the proposition had been referred, had met immediately after the Council meeting at which it had been accepted, and previous discussion enabled the Committee at once to consider in detail the style of gowns for Members and Fellows, with hats to match. Messrs Ede and Ravenscroft were appointed robe makers to the College.

All this was reported at the next Council meeting on 9th April 1926, at which sample gowns were available for inspection. President Clarkson said: "May I . . . ask for volunteers as mannequins?" Councillors Bradley and McKinna obliged. It was then agreed "that the Council resolve itself into Committee for exhibition for the gowns."

On Friday 7th January 1927 the RCVS Council for the first time met in academic dress.

In the 1920's, then, there was professional progress on many fronts. When the Annual Dinner was under discussion at the RCVS Council meeting on 9th January 1925, with twenty-nine Councillors present, it is recorded that: "A show of hands was taken for the purpose of deciding whether ladies should be invited, and it was decided that they should not, only three voting for."

Here, again, was progress. A decade earlier no vote would have been taken, it being already known that all would be against.

CHAPTER 18

Veterinary research and the Agricultural Research Council

An account has been given of the development of veterinary education in Ireland, to the point at which a teaching school was opened in Dublin in 1900 with Mettam as Principal. The school prospered under his guidance, in spite of financial problems that were common to all British veterinary schools at the time.

Mettam died in November 1917, and was succeeded as Principal by Scotsman J.F. Craig, who had joined the Dublin staff in 1903 to teach anatomy, and five years later had been elected Professor of Medicine and Parasitology. He was a man of vigorous intellect, who played an important part in preserving the connection between the Dublin school and the RCVS after creation of the Irish Free State in December 1921, proclaimed officially a year later.

Lack of urgency was a feature of negotiations to adjust the association of the RCVS with a Dublin school now outside the United Kingdom. Indeed, April 1925 had been reached before the RCVS wrote to the Colonial Office "calling attention to the necessity for an official ruling with regard to the relationship of the Royal College to members practising in the Irish Free State, and to students in training at the Royal Veterinary College of Ireland." In answer to this enquiry, it was explained that "under the present state of the law the Veterinary Surgeons' Acts did not apply to the Free State." At a meeting of the RCVS Council on 3rd July 1925, Principal Craig of Dublin was "happy . . . to know that the bulk of the profession in Ireland are earnest in their desire that the present relationship with the Royal College shall continue," and he believed that "the State is not averse to that idea." He asked for, and was unanimously given, an assurance that the RCVS had "no intention of altering . . . or severing . . . connection with Ireland."

In January 1927 the Irish Free State Sub-Committee of the RCVS, formed to deal with further negotiations, was told by Principal Craig that

298 of 320 members of the Veterinary Medical Association of Ireland had "supported the recommendations of the Council that the Veterinary Surgeons Acts should be adapted by the Irish Free State Government to the Irish Free State." This clear majority in favour of continuing an association between the RCVS and the profession in the Irish Free State, resulted in approval in April 1929 by the RCVS Council of drafts of an Irish Free State Veterinary Surgeons Act, and of a Supplemental Charter to provide for election to the Council of "four representatives of the members residing in the Irish Free State, in addition to the present 32 members."

The Veterinary Surgeons (Irish Free State Agreement) Act received Royal Assent on 17th March 1932, and the Supplemental Charter was royally approved three weeks later. Irish representatives (elected in the Irish Free State) Craig, Dolan, Donnelly and Dodd, joined the RCVS Council on 1st July 1932, to a warm welcome from President Male and "prolonged applause."

*　　*　　*

In 1928 and 1929 two Governmental Reports were published on exclusively veterinary matters. The first (in November 1928) was by the Lovat Committee appointed in July 1927 by the Secretary of State for the Colonies to examine veterinary research and administration in the non-self-governing Dependencies. The second (in August 1929) was of the Martin Committee appointed in July 1928 by the Minister of Agriculture and Fisheries to consider reconstruction of the Royal Veterinary College (i.e. the London teaching school).

Both Reports expressed dissatisfaction, and were timely stimuli to an administration indifferent to veterinary matters. It must be emphasised, however, that they merely echoed what had been said for years, and said, and said again, by the profession, collectively through its schools and the RCVS, and individually by such men as Hunting, McFadyean, Stockman, and Bradley, about inadequate Government support for veterinary science. This emphasis is necessary because of a belief that was once general, and has not yet been obliterated, that veterinary surgeons are incapable of knowing their own business and that for full expression of their talents, they require advice from doctors of medicine, professors of the purer sciences, upper-echelon administrators, and landed laymen.

The Lovat Committee found that Britain had "done little for tropical veterinary science." Veterinary departments were "in general neglected and under-staffed." There were "only 127 qualified officers in the Service, or one to every 16,000 square miles, 400,000 inhabitants, or

280,000 head of stock." There was no advisory authority at the Colonial Office, no coherent administration, no coordinated research. The "general policy" was "one of drift." Succinct proposals covered recruitment, training, and conditions of service, and included creation of scholarships to enable science graduates to train as veterinary surgeons, on the understanding that they would enter the Colonial Veterinary Service for at least three years. An Adviser on Animal Health was to be appointed to the Colonial Office. Implementation, in the fullness of time, of most of this Committee's proposals, enhanced the quality of the veterinary services overseas.

The Martin Committee revealed the dilapidation of the London school, the premier veterinary teaching establishment in Britain and the Empire. It found the work "being carried on under conditions which are a national disgrace . . . the end of the current year will find the College devoid of all reserves with its prospective income insufficient to cover essential expenditure . . . the pass to which affairs have been brought has not been due to any lack of enthusiasm . . . of the Governing body . . . or to the small staff, who despite their meagre salaries and wholly inadequate facilities, continued loyally at their work. It is nothing less than extraordinary that the College has been able, in spite of the most depressing circumstances, to turn out year by year a regular flow of qualified students."

The recommendations of this Committee were precise. The school must be rebuilt on the existing site, and re-equipped to provide accommodation for 250 students, and a yearly intake of seventy-five. London, "with its vast population, ensuring the maintenance of adequate clinical material," was preferable to "a rural site," and offered the prospect of University affiliation. A capital grant from the Government of £300,000 was recommended, together with £21,000 and £4,500 annually for maintenance and Departmental research, respectively. The maintenance grant for the Research Institute at the school should be "substantially increased," and the "Institute should also be provided with a field station in the vicinity of London for the purpose of experimental work with the larger animals." The government of the school should be revised under a new Charter.

McFadyean gave evidence to the Martin Committee, although he had retired in 1927. The similarity is remarkable between the Martin Report and the cumulative minutes of meetings of the school's Governors and its General Purposes Committee during the thirty-three years of McFadyean's Principalship. The Report was consummation of a dream.

Government found itself unable to spare all the money recommended, but £100,000 would be made available for rebuilding provided the school raised a similar sum. This was achieved by Principal Hobday, who had followed McFadyean, and the rebuilt school was opened by King George VI and Queen Elizabeth on 9th November 1937.

*   *   *

McFadyean was President of the RCVS for the years 1906–09. In 1930 that honour was again conferred on him, for the special reason that the Eleventh International Veterinary Congress was to be held in London that year, and he was to be its President. The profession wished him to represent them not only personally, but also as leader of their governing body. This Congress would be the first since the ill-fated gathering in London in the first week of August 1914, with McFadyean President, abruptly abandoned as war broke out. The clock had moved on sixteen years. Colleagues in peace had been enemies in war. Now a common veterinary cause brought together 1,800 from sixty nations, again in London, again with McFadyean in the Presidential Chair. At seventy-seven, he was an international father figure, and he led that great assembly with characteristic courtesy and command.

In his Presidential Address, McFadyean recalled the history of international veterinary meetings. The first, with an attendance of 101, was in Hamburg in 1863, convened by John Gamgee, "one of the best informed and most enlightened members of the veterinary profession . . . at that time." Gamgee foresaw value in discussions among veterinary surgeons from different countries on "the increasing prevalence of contagious disease amongst cattle, sheep and other farm animals . . . and the consequent necessity of advising Governments to prevent export of such animals from one country to another." The first international pooling of veterinary experience set the pattern for further meetings. Vienna 1865, Zurich 1867, Brussels 1883, Paris 1889, Berne 1895, Baden-Baden 1899, Budapest 1905, the Hague 1909, London 1914. Up to the time of the Congress in Budapest "all the subjects had been discussed in general meeting one at a time," but with over 1,000 people attending it became obvious that there would have to be specialist sections, in addition to plenary sessions. After the Budapest Congress a Permanent Commission was established, with representatives from several countries, so that continuity was maintained from congress to congress.

That first post-war Congress in London in 1930 concentrated into a few days the strides in veterinary science over two decades since the last full Congress in the Hague. For men of McFadyean's generation, the world of their youth was well-nigh unbelievable. Had there *really* been a time before the tubercle bacillus? Younger men caught the excitement of progress since those far-off days. Rancour and the strains of war had disappeared.

The Congress Banquet was held at the Connaught Rooms, Great Queen Street, London, on 7th August. When the formal toasts were over, when talk and reminiscence had had their generous sway, and the hour was growing late, McFadyean rose to bring a splendid evening to its close. He saw everywhere, he said, distinguished men from many lands; without hypocrisy they could be assured: "This is one of the proudest moments of my life."

A proud moment, certainly, but two other proud occasions were to follow. In 1933 McFadyean was elected first Honorary Fellow of the RCVS. The Supplemental Charter of 1932 had been obtained essentially to provide for election to the RCVS Council of representatives of the profession from the Irish Free State (already described), but the opportunity had been taken to cover a few other matters, among which was election of Members of long-standing to Fellowship of the RCVS for outstanding service to the profession. Immediately this franchise was granted, the RCVS Council unanimously nominated John McFadyean its first Fellow by election. The date of this nomination was 19th April 1932, the fifty-seventh anniversary of his graduation from the Edinburgh veterinary school. In presenting this unique Fellowship at the RCVS Annual General Meeting on 7th June 1933, President Buxton said: "Who am I to put into words those sentiments that express the devotion of the profession for the very name McFadyean?"

"The devotion of the profession" was felicitously "put into words" four years later, however, when the quarterly *Journal of Comparative Pathology and Therapeutics* reached the fiftieth annual volume, every issue having been personally edited by McFadyean. It was an extraordinary achievement by any standard, but against the background of his other preoccupations it was miraculous. It meant that for half-a-century, wherever he might have been, whatever his other commitments, he had had manuscripts to read, authors to consult, printers to advise, proofs to check, editorials, annotations, abstracts to write, and, of course, his own unceasing researches to prepare for publication. As 1937 drew near, he was persuaded to allow colleagues to produce the final number of the fiftieth volume of his *Journal* as a *Festschrift*, a personal tribute from grateful readers across the world. It was published on 31st December 1937, and right royally did it reflect a proud occasion. Photographs, original articles, reprinted material from writings and speeches, personal tributes, anecdotes and recollections. It is unique in British veterinary literature.

*   *   *

To Major-General Sir Frederick Smith, who died in July 1929, the veterinary profession was — literally — life. Son of an Army quartermaster who died on service in India, Fred Smith knew the pinch of poverty in London from his earliest days, and owed his education to the Royal Patriotic Fund. He entered the London veterinary school in October 1873, and during his student days developed a regimen for frugal living and mental discipline that intensified as he grew older. RCVS Secretary Bullock, with whom, in later years, he was closely associated, recorded that Smith "neglected every social duty . . . rose at 5 a.m., and with but two breaks for meals, a breakfast and a dinner, his waking hours were spent at work of some kind." His life in India was "just as strenuous as at home; he never visited a hill station, even in the hot weather; he was too busy working in the plains. He abstained from alcohol, and drank nothing but water." In an obituary in his *Journal*, McFadyean wrote: "Sir Frederick held stern views of life and duty . . . inspired by a determination to contribute his utmost to the advancement of veterinary science . . . his plan of work did not leave him even the minimum of time necessary for rest and recreation if health is to be preserved."

This dedication brought promotion in 1907 to the most senior post in the Army Veterinary Service, and was expressed in numerous scientific papers, text-books on Veterinary Hygiene and Veterinary Physiology, a veterinary history of the South African war, a history of the Royal Army Veterinary Corps, and "The Early History of Veterinary Literature and its British Development," being an account, in four volumes, of veterinary literature from antiquity to 1866.

Clearly, anyone seeking information on British veterinary history must turn first to Major-General Smith. In this present history, original sources were compared with Smith's observations on veterinary people of the late eighteenth and the nineteenth centuries, and it was realised, with dismay, that some of Smith's conclusions, emphatically stated, did not apparently tally with the facts. Smith's dismissal of James Beart Simonds as historically insignificant has already been noted, but other individuals — some praised, some blamed — might equally be re-assessed.

Two points are pertinent. First, Bullock, whose admiration and affection for Smith are beyond question, wrote of him: "He was . . . not always right in judging the character of some of those with whom he had to work."

This failing was strangely in contrast with the unusually keen powers of observation and logical deduction he displayed in his work." Secondly, Volume IV of "The Early History of Veterinary Literature and its British Development" (covering the period 1824 – 1866), was published more than three years after Smith's death, from manuscript entrusted to Bullock. In a Preface, Bullock explained that when preparing the manuscript, Smith (then in his seventies) was unable, because of poor health, "to travel to London to make use of the Library of the College or of the British Museum and had to rely on information sent to him by correspondents in answer to specific questions." Bullock added that: "No attempt has been made to modify any of the author's expressions of opinion." In a biographical note on Smith in that final volume, Bullock described the manner in which the manuscript had been completed: "A severe attack of cardiac asthma in May, 1928, warned him that his end was near. He took the warning seriously, gave up his house and retired to furnished rooms. There, under great and increasing difficulties, he continued to struggle with his literary work, up to within a few days of his death."

Historical evaluation may have been distorted by this fight, in shrinking time, to complete too great a task.

* * *

It has been noted that the Report in 1922 of the Advisory Committee on Research into Diseases of Animals, recommended extensive support, through the Development Commission, for veterinary research, and that soon afterwards the windfall of the Corn Repeal Fund provided the necessary money. Research institutes were established in London and Cambridge, there was Government backing for the Animal Diseases Research Association in Scotland, and extended support for the veterinary laboratories of the Ministry of Agriculture and Fisheries at Weybridge. However, the manner of controlling these funds had still to be agreed. Discussion was initiated by a recommendation in the 1922 Report to establish an advisory "Diseases of Animals Research Committee" to allocate funds, but McFadyean opposed this in a minority comment, preferring direct negotiation between research laboratories and the Development Commission.

The case for coordination of veterinary research in the United Kingdom, was brought to the attention of the body of the profession by Major-General Sir John Moore, F.R.C.V.S., first as a resolution accepted by the Central Veterinary Society "that there should be set up a Diseases of Animals Research Council or Board," and, shortly afterwards, in an article in *The Veterinary Record* of 31st March 1923. Moore believed that veterinary research should be administered by a body similar to the Medical Research Council, or "be co-opted into one common Government Department of Scientific Research." Indeed, he was so obsessed by the necessity for central control of veterinary research, that in *The Veterinary Record* of 2nd June 1923 he maintained that if control could not be via "one large organisation of State," then a "Council should be separately constituted and incorporated by Royal Charter under the administrative direction of a Committee of the Privy Council." With more enthusiasm than tact, he actually named a "Diseases of Animals Research Council," of which he himself would be "General Secretary (*pro tem.*)," supported by "Assistant Secretary, Publications and Controller of Records (£500 per annum); Clerk of Accounts (£250)." The veterinary members of his team were to be McFadyean, Stockman, Sumner, Bradley, Brittlebank, Buxton, Gaiger, and Craig.

No record has been found of the reactions of these gentlemen to his fantasy.

The handful of veterinary surgeons involved in research at that time were unequivocally opposed to being organised by a committee. This was made clear at a meeting of the RCVS Council on 8th January 1926 in response to Councillor Sir John Moore's proposal: "That sanction be obtained for the creation of an official veterinary research council in Great Britain." He said: "I feel a certain amount of trepidation, for two reasons. One is that I am not a research officer, nor can I claim to be very intimately associated with research. The second is that there are perhaps several members of the Council who do not quite agree with the resolution I have proposed . . . my sole desire is to . . . advance our profession." At some length, he then repeated the proposition, summarised above, that he had been canvassing for three years.

Councillor Chief Veterinary Officer Stockman, unable to attend this meeting, asked the Council to accept a letter *in lieu* of a personal statement, because of his vital concern with Moore's proposal. He wrote: "My feeling about these Committees and Councils is that they are a disease of the age. I, like many others, have suffered in my work from being Committee-ridden . . . at their best, one finds these Committees composed largely of men who are not in the fighting-line of research . . . long Reports have to be prepared . . . for no particular purpose . . . except that the Committee exists. Personally, I am dead against any such body as Sir John Moore proposes." Stockman added that he found that veterinary research was satisfactorily controlled by the existing Council for Agricultural Research covered by the Development Commission.

Supporting Stockman's point of view, McFadyean was "unable to recognise . . . what exactly was going to be the benefit of this new research council." He said: "It would be for myself a terrifying prospect that any committee should be appointed to interfere with or endeavour to control the work which is carried out in the institute with which I am connected . . . in my opinion this motion should be disposed of immediately . . . the Development Commission has itself an advisory committee, and the Ministry of Agriculture has a committee of which all the heads of the institutes that are receiving grants from the Development Fund are members. We meet periodically . . . the present position . . . is eminently satisfactory."

The discussion continued, in gentlemanly fashion, with Sir John Moore retreating gallantly. Eventually, he had to concede defeat.

Stockman died a few months after this meeting, however, and McFadyean retired the following year. The Lovat and Martin Committees reported in 1928 and 1929 respectively. Veterinary research was expanding rapidly, no longer exclusively motivated by dedicated individuals. Government finance, and scholarships based on schools and institutes, were creating a new breed of full-time specialists in research techniques, attracted as much by stimulating work and reasonable remuneration, as by the intellectual challenge that transcends all worldly matters. Co-ordination of their activities was inevitable.

In its issue for 18th October 1930, *The Veterinary Record* reported that: "An Agricultural Research Council is being constituted to secure improved co-ordination and extension of agricultural research throughout the United Kingdom . . . we await with interest the announcement of the names of the members of the veterinary profession who will be nominated to serve on the Council."

A grenade was thrown in the House of Commons on 6th July 1931 by Dr Addison, Minister of Agriculture and Fisheries, when the names were announced of the thirteen members of the new Agricultural Research Council, created a body corporate under a Charter by Order in Council dated 29th June 1931. The shattered *Veterinary Record* of 18th July commented: "It will be a great surprise to readers to note that though bacteriologists of the medical profession, biologists, mycologists and biochemists have been selected for appointment, not a single veterinary expert has been included." The *Record* struggled to be objective about the men described by the Minister as "appointed either on account of their qualifications in one or other of the basic sciences underlying agriculture, or on account of their general experience of and interest in agriculture." Hot indignation could not be concealed, however, that the profession had been excluded from decision-making on matters so specifically veterinary as research on bovine tuberculosis, foot-and-mouth disease, contagious abortion, swine fever and other farm-livestock diseases.

Omission of a veterinary surgeon from that first Agricultural Research Council reawakened the resentments of earlier years, and came perilously close to rule by clique. A letter from Sir John Moore in *The Times* of 13th July 1931 regretted the Minister's decision, and a week later in the same newspaper, with a pen honed for years, Sir John McFadyean averred: "The public affront which has thus been put upon the veterinary profession will be deeply resented by all its members."

A gesture towards the profession was made by the Agricultural Research Council early in 1932, when Sir John Moore and R.E. Montgomery, Animal Health Adviser to the Colonial Office, were co-opted to an animal diseases survey committee. Montgomery, a retired Colonial veterinary officer, died a few months later, however, and Moore, now sixty-eight, had spent his life with Army horses. It was a palliative gesture, therefore, rather than a serious attempt to obtain the best available advice on diseases of farm animals.

This ungracious attitude of the Agricultural Research Council continued into 1934. Gradually, however, a few veterinary surgeons were woven into a network of 'Standing,' 'Other,' and 'Special' committees. By December of that year *The Veterinary Record* could express cautious general approval, while continuing to deplore the absence from the Council itself, now in its fourth year, of a veterinary surgeon. That appointment came eventually in February 1936 when, in answer to a question in the House of Commons, the Lord President of the Council, Mr Ramsay MacDonald, announced that the Agricultural Research Council was to "be strengthened" by addition to its ranks of "Mr John Smith, O.B.E., M.R.C.V.S., D.V.H., formerly Director of Animal Health in Northern Rhodesia," The profession made the required congratulatory noises, but wondered why a retired colonial administrator had been preferred to a younger man with British experience, of whom several of outstanding ability were available.

In a back room at the Agricultural Research Council's offices in 6[a] Dean's Yard, Westminster, however, someone, for some time, had had a genuine interest in veterinary research, in spite of official proclivity to keep the profession at arm's length. In May 1937 *The Veterinary Record* reported that: "The Agricultural Research Council are negotiating for the purchase of Mr Alfred Barclay's dairy farm at Compton, Berkshire, where they propose to conduct large-scale experiments in the elimination and prevention of cattle diseases." This farm had been chosen because the cattle were "widely known for their milking qualities and freedom from disease."

Purchase of the Compton Manor Estate of 1,500 acres in Berkshire was announced in *The Veterinary Record* of 23rd October 1937. The Director was to be G.W. Dunkin, M.R.C.V.S., recently associated with Patrick Ladilaw at the Medical Research Council's laboratories at Mill Hill in classic experiments on dog distemper, that had resulted in a protective vaccine. *The Veterinary Record* said: "We have not hesitated in the past to criticise the Agricultural Research Council . . ." but ". . . we offer . . . sincere congratulations upon the step which they have taken. It is one of the most significant moves in the history of veterinary research in this country."

CHAPTER 19

Sulphonamides, vaccines, metabolic disease. A State service

A good deal has been said about the development of veterinary research in Britain, from the Pasteur/Koch era of the 1880's to the third decade of the twentieth century. A slow, slow beginning was followed by awakening interest in the 1920's, and in the 1930's by eager research throughout the Kingdom. In explanation of apparent omission of the veterinary surgeon in general practice from this story, it is emphasised that understanding of the causes and pathology of diseases far outstripped prevention and treatment. If veterinary practice of 1935 be compared, disease for disease, with that of 1905, similarities are greater than differences. Veterinary father and son rolled pills and folded powders from ingredients bought in bulk. Turpentine was a stand-by medicament, as also were liquid paraffin and castor oil, aloes, too, and common salt, soapy-water enemas, iodine for wounds, and carbolic acid for disinfection.

In three respects, however, the veterinary practitioner of the 1930's was on the verge of new pastures.

First, a drug that would attack 'blood-poisoning' micro-organisms, the streptococci, was discovered in 1935 at the I.G. Farben Industrie laboratories in Germany. It was named 'Prontosil,' and its efficacy was demonstrated at the Queen Charlotte Hospital in London in 1936 by successful treatment of the frequently fatal puerperal fever of women. The antibacterial ingredient of 'Prontosil' was found to be sulphonamide, the first of a series of similar compounds that were active against a range of hitherto untreatable human and animal diseases.

Secondly, vaccines against several important diseases of farm livestock were coming into general use. Thus, by the mid-1930's the sheep diseases braxy, lamb-dysentery, and louping-ill were largely under control by vaccines, following research by the Animal Diseases Research Association in Scotland, the Wellcome laboratories at Beckenham, and the Institute of Animal Pathology in Cambridge. The possibility of field control of disease by artificial immunisation had been demonstrated, of course, by Pasteur's classic experiment with anthrax in 1881, but production of artificial immunity against many other infectious diseases had posed problems that were insoluble without research. Suitable research facilities were not available in Britain until well into the twentieth century.

Thirdly, a simple and efficient treatment became available for milk fever in the cow, a common and often fatal disease feared by every dairy farmer. Milk fever plagued veterinary practitioners for years, and the story of its control and understanding is an unusual blend of empiricism and astute research, that pointed to hitherto unsuspected diseases caused by defective metabolism.

Milk fever was named before invention of the clinical thermometer. There is, in fact, no fever, and 'post-parturient paresis' would be more appropriate, if that name were likely to be understood. Milk fever it was at the beginning, however, and will always be. Fever is absent, but there is certainly a relationship with milk-production. Characteristically, the disease occurs within a few hours of calving, when the mammary gland is heavy with milk for the newborn calf. The cow sways, collapses suddenly, and lies helpless, often with head turned towards a flank. Dullness develops, quickly, followed in a few hours by coma, that is the prelude to death. Timing of the various stages of the disease can very widely, but in the absence of treatment prognosis is poor.

Milk fever was not overlooked in the scramble to match microorganisms with diseases, that followed Koch's discovery of the tubercle bacillus in 1882. Disease after disease yielded its special microbe, but not milk fever. Affected cows were bled, blistered, purged, starved, milked out, left unmilked, and given every potion, to no avail. Some died. Some recovered. Many were butchered, the flesh to be eaten to lessen the loss.

In 1902 McFadyean's *Journal* published, in translation, a remarkable paper by Danish veterinary surgeon Jürgens Schmidt, entitled: "The Development of the Treatment of Milk Fever During the Last Five Years." As the cause of milk fever was unknown, Schmidt had treated symptoms, and had attempted in one case to reduce swelling in the udder by injecting via the milk canals in the teats a litre of a solution of potassium iodide in water, massaging the fluid throughout the gland. To his astonishment, there was marked general clinical improvement within a few hours. Colleagues confirmed Schmidt's observation, but did not understand — any more than he did — why an innocuous chemical in weak solution should have so marked an effect.

The puzzle was then twisted oddly. A veterinary surgeon called to a case of milk fever, discovered that his potassium iodide solution had been left at home. Understandably wishing to avoid loss of face, he injected water into the udder, and said he would return shortly to see the patient again, intending on the second visit to give the correct injection of potassium iodide. However, by the time he returned he was amazed to find that the cow had responded to the injection of water as if to potassium iodide. It was clear, then, that the injection *per se* had caused the clinical improvement.

Schmidt continued the story in his paper of 1902. Veterinary surgeon Andersen pumped air instead of water into the udder of a milk fever case, postulating that increased pressure within the udder was the critical factor. His guess was correct, and the result dramatic. Recoveries from milk fever became commonplace, and Schmidt was now able to report 884 successes in 914 cases treated by inflation of the udder, with an average period of just over six hours between pumping air into an apparently dying cow and that animal standing up of her own accord and turning hungrily to the manger. The foreign veterinary press was briefly sceptical, but the efficacy of this unlikely treatment was soon confirmed everywhere. Schmidt had pondered deeply on the matter, and in that paper of 1902 he made the prescient suggestion that artificially increased pressure within the udder reduced milk secretion and blood supply, thereby halting the sudden post-calving drain on the dam's metabolic resources.

At this point the problem should have been handed to veterinary biochemists for further investigation, but none such existed in 1902. For over twenty years there was no advance in knowledge of milk fever. In 1925, however, Dryerre and Greig of the Edinburgh veterinary school suggested that the cause might be a sudden loss of body calcium. They agreed with Schmidt's hypothesis that air pumped into the udder reduced the blood supply and flow of milk, and they added that the net effect was to prevent loss from the body of vital calcium. This hypothesis was examined in several laboratories, and by 1928 was considered likely to be correct. In the meantime, Dryerre and Greig had been successfully treating milk fever by subcutaneous injection of salts of calcium, although, unfortunately, many of these injections caused nasty local reactions.

The practical difficulties at that time of research on large farm animals are emphasised by a comment in one of Dryerre and Greig's papers: "An . . . obstacle was . . . the reluctance of veterinary practitioners to experiment with a hitherto untried treatment, when one of almost specific efficacy, that of mammary inflation, was in their hands. After considerable difficulty, we, however, eventually obtained the services of a firm of insurance agents who were prepared to effect a special form of insurance to cover the value of cases of milk fever experimentally treated by calcium therapy."

The problem of local reaction to injection of calcium salts was solved partly by Dryerre and Greig, and partly by the American Hayden working at Cornell. The former found that gluconate of calcium was much less irritant than other salts, and the latter reported that boric acid was a powerful solvent for calcium gluconate. These observations combined to produce a highly active, readily injectable remedy for milk fever — calcium boro-gluconate. Of course, inflation of the udder would still do the trick, but it cannot be overlooked that a hypodermic syringe has a more professional image than a bicycle pump.

*   *   *

After early irritation had been pardoned, co-ordination of veterinary research at schools and institutes by the Agricultural Research Council was accepted as helpful to research workers and their administrators. Staff of the Ministry of Agriculture and Fisheries were outside this arrangement, however, and development of this branch of the profession must now be considered.

In 1932 an Economic Advisory Council Committee on Cattle Diseases was appointed by the Prime Minister, with Sir Gowland Hopkins as Chairman. The objective was to examine the incidence of diseases of cattle, with special reference to tuberculosis and the production of disease-free milk, and to consider whether changes in administrative practice were required to control these diseases.

The Committee's Report of 16th April 1934 set in motion far-reaching reorganisation of the British State Veterinary Service. It was recommended that local authorities should be obliged to provide routine veterinary inspection of all herds and dairies, and that this greatly expanded service should be supervised by the Ministry of Agriculture and Fisheries. Control of bovine tuberculosis was the immediate objective, with complete eradication the ultimate goal. In addition to an incidence of bovine tuberculosis approaching forty per cent, the Report revealed unexpectedly high figures for Johne's disease, contagious abortion, and mastitis, and the necessity was obvious for concerted action.

Encouraged by this Report, the National Veterinary Medical Association (NVMA) set up a committee "to frame proposals showing how the services of the veterinary profession can best be utilised."

Parenthetically, it is emphasised that this investigation was initiated by the NVMA, not the RCVS, indicating the extent to which the former organisation had by this time assumed the role of political watch-dog for the profession.

The NVMA committee's conclusions were published on 25th April 1936. A Department of Animal Health should be established, of which the Principal Veterinary Officer should be directly responsible to the Minister of State. Beneath him should be Area, County, Municipal, and Laboratory Veterinary Officers. There should be panels of practitioners to assist the full-time officers, and there should be area laboratories. There were recommendations on the method of appointing officers, and on their accountability within the organisation.

The Veterinary Record of 5th June 1937 assured the profession that the NVMA proposals had been widely canvassed by "not infrequent deputations that have waited upon the Ministry and other influential bodies," and that they appeared "likely to be implemented." Legislation to co-ordinate the work of veterinary surgeons variously employed by the Ministry of Agriculture and Fisheries, the Department of Agriculture for Scotland, and local authorities over the whole country, was covered by the Agriculture Bill 1937, before Parliament in July 1937. *The Veterinary Record* of 10th July rejoiced that "the Government's intentions follow closely the scheme put forward by the National Veterinary Medical Association," and hoped that "co-ordination of the veterinary services, including practitioners and several specialised branches . . . may be brought into being."

The profession's rejoicing was short-lived. Five months later *The Veterinary Record* expressed concern over secret discussions about a centralised veterinary service, details of which were "gradually filtering through to the profession from non-professional sources," and in an editorial entitled "Disillusion," dated Christmas Day 1937, stated bluntly: "Unfortunately, the counsel of the profession has not truly been sought, its consultative committee has been presented with defined schemes in which it has been expected to acquiesce almost at once. A policy of secrecy, a spirit suggestive of dictatorship and an apparent assumption of omniscience have prevailed."

It was a repetition of the Agricultural Research Council's early days. Veterinary surgeons were instructed, not consulted.

The NVMA Council held an emergency meeting on 23rd December 1937, to receive the report of a special committee that had been attempting to put the profession's views to Mr W.S. Morrison, Minister of Agriculture and Fisheries, before final decisions were made on the organisation of a centralised veterinary service — "the greatest potential development the profession has experienced this century." The Minister

had refused to receive a deputation, giving his reasons "in a long letter
. . . that seriously misinterprets many points in the President's letter
dated December 15th." This was childish and churlish, and *The Veterinary Record* of 1st January 1938 had reason to comment: "This profession has worked steadfastly for years towards the establishment of a co-
ordinated service to combat the diseases of animals, and it is a bitter disappointment . . . to see the hopes which had arisen with the introduction
of the Agriculture Act gradually expelled."

The NVMA continued to press for an interview with the Minister.
They were refused three times.

Then the olive twig, and all honour to the man who offered it.

On 29th January 1938, with unfeigned relief, *The Veterinary Record*
reported that: "Sir Donald Fergusson — the Permanent Secretary to the
Ministry — has asked some members of the Consultative Committee of
the Association to . . . discuss frankly the present situation."

Once discussion was started, the breakneck speed of reconciliation
indicated that the Ministry had indeed been listening to the profession,
but had been unwilling to admit the merit of its proposals. Negotiations
for a mutually acceptable scheme were completed in two months, no less.

The Animal Health Division of the Ministry of Agriculture and
Fisheries came into being on 1st April 1938. Its organisation was virtually
that proposed by the NVMA two years previously. Twenty-two areas
embracing seventy-eight divisions covered the whole country. Veterinary
surgeons in practice assisted their full-time colleagues, at first as a temporary measure, but later permanently when their essential contribution
was recognised. At last it had become realistic to envisage eradication of
tuberculosis, and control, through nationwide co-operation, of other
farm livestock diseases.

*   *   *

The tale has been told to 1886 of the search for adequate headquarters
for the RCVS. In that year occupation was taken of a new building at
No. 10 Red Lion Square, erected on the site of a previous house of which
the freehold had been purchased to permit demolition and reconstruction. It has been mentioned that the new building was erected so quickly
that there was not even time to observe the Foundation Stone ritual.

High-speed construction probably explains why Councillor Mc-
Fadyean referred to "this rotten old building," at a meeting of the RCVS
Council on 12th July 1919 (only thirty-three years later), and why the
Council was unanimous that "immensely better accommodation" was
required. As so often in the history of the RCVS, however, lack of funds

prevented action. Installation of central heating in 1922 was a minor concession to comfort, and the following year a sub-committee probed defective acoustics in the Council Chamber, taking a deal of trouble to experiment with curtains, screens, and rearrangement of furniture and seating. In 1927 inadequate accommodation was again, and with irritation, discussed, and two years later, in preparation for a possible move, a valuation was made of the building and its contents, at £12,000 and £5,800 respectively.

Again and again, however, more adequate accommodation was beyond the RCVS purse. By 1933 it was not safe to have meetings in the library on the second floor, because of the addition of the weight of people to that of books, and in desperation, but without success, Secretary Bullock sought extra space at No. 9 next door. Acquisition of new premises was now top priority. The Finance Committee reported in April 1934: "The building at 10 Red Lion Square . . . consists of two offices, a Council Room and a Library. There is no convenient room for committee meetings, there is no waiting-room, there is no room to house the outflow from the rapidly expanding library . . . the task of finding a convenient building to fit the special requirements of the College will not be easy."

Action at almost any price was essential. An Additional Accommodation Committee was formed in June 1935, "to enter into negotiations with regard to the adjacent properties in Red Lion Square, and make further enquiries in other districts." Shortly afterwards, a letter was received by the RCVS from the NVMA (also in search of more suitable accommodation) "on the question of . . . combining to secure premises for housing both bodies." A joint meeting on 8th January 1936 politely lacked enthusiasm, but agreed to bear in mind the possibility of shared premises if a really suitable site were found. In the event, the RCVS decided to develop its existing site, and was about to accept architects' plans when, in January 1937, a letter was received from Mr Davis the owner of No. 9 Red Lion Square "stating that he was now able to offer the whole of the freehold premises." The scheme for enlargement of No. 10 was abandoned forthwith, and the freehold of No. 9 was purchased for £10,000.

There were many besides Secretary Bullock who wished that Mr Davis had been less coy, wasting a massive amount of their time for several years.

Within a few months of this satisfactory ending of the RCVS search, the NVMA also found "quarters more in keeping both as to address and accommodation with the requirements of a national body representative of British veterinary interests throughout the Empire." They moved from "life in rooms" at 2 Verulam Buildings, Gray's Inn, to "a handsome, spacious building" at 36 Gordon Square.

*   *   *

It will be recalled that both William Hunting's *Veterinary Record* and John McFadyean's *Journal of Comparative Pathology and Therapeutics* were launched in 1888. The golden jubilee *Festschrift* of the latter has been described. The jubilee number of *The Veterinary Record* of 16th July 1938 carried a widely-ranging historical tribute from the Editorial Committee, written by J.T. Edwards. The *Record's* achievement was as great in the field of domestic journalism as was that of McFadyean's scientific *Journal*, and it is a source of wonder that not once in fifty years was it overwhelmed by the pressure of weekly publication. Continuous topicality and high ethical and literary standards stimulated and gave common purpose to the members of an emerging profession.

The *Record* was vital to the development of the NVMA, of which it became the mouthpiece in 1921. It is to the credit of the new editors that, overall, they maintained Hunting's objective to report for the whole profession. Meetings of the NVMA Council and of its Divisions were given prominence, of course, but RCVS Council meetings were fully recorded, and opinions at variance with NVMA policies were fairly expressed. It is true that as the influence of the NVMA increased in the 1920's and 1930's some editorials seemed to infer that the NVMA controlled the profession, but these exceptions reflected exuberance of individual leader-writers, rather than intention to lessen the authority of the RCVS. By 1938 Hunting's twelve pages of 1888 had become forty, handsomely printed on glossy paper, but the objectives were the same — to inform, instruct and publicise the whole profession.

*   *   *

Within months of the Munich Agreement of September 1938, war seemed inevitable. Veterinary surgeons wished information on the care of animals if conflict came. The great unknown was attack by air. *The Veterinary Record* tried to help. On 24th June 1939 it said: "Measures for the protection of the human populace in the event of raids by hostile aircraft have been under consideration for some years . . . it is with anxiety that we of the veterinary profession view the paucity of official measures designed to protect animals." The NVMA had been pressing for Government Air Raid Precautions (ARP) action for over two years, and by invitation of the Home Secretary a Departmental Committee with representatives from the Ministry of Agriculture, the Royal Army Veterinary Corps, the RCVS and the NVMA met in January 1938. It was talk with little action, however, and the *Record* now warned the profession that in spite of efforts by the NVMA and the RSPCA: "The public . . . still remains largely oblivious to the need for ARP measures for animals." It urged "individual veterinary surgeons . . . to stimulate their local authorities."

At the outbreak of war there was no plan for the special use of veterinary surgeons. The requirements of the Royal Army Veterinary Corps, and the liability of veterinary surgeons and students for military service were discussed on 11th September 1939, when the Presidents of the RCVS and the NVMA, the Secretary of the RCVS and the Deputy Chief Veterinary Officer met the Director of the Army Veterinary Services at the War Office. *The Veterinary Record* of 16th September advised that: "Members . . . will serve the national interest best by remaining in their appointments or practice until a . . . statement is published." In due course, veterinary surgeons were designated members of a reserved occupation. *The Veterinary Record* of 22nd June 1940 commented enigmatically: "For reasons which we are still unable to disclose, the Ministry of Agriculture and other Government Departments have foreseen circumstances in which the entire personnel of the veterinary profession may become fully occupied in safe-guarding the livestock of the nation."

By mid-May 1940, with German armies smashing towards the French coast, air-borne invasion of the British mainland appeared imminent. *The Veterinary Record* of 18th May relayed an official request: "To keep an unremitting vigilance on any incidents which may appear . . . suspicious . . . the veterinary surgeon in the pursuit of his professional duties by day and by night, together with his intimate knowledge of the countryside, is particularly capable of acquiring information which may prove of exceptional value to the Authorities."

At the beginning of June 1940 the veterinary profession in Britain received by cablegram a generous invitation, addressed to Secretary Bullock of the RCVS: "Members of Ontario Veterinary Association desire you to convey to veterinarians in Great Britain, those contemplating evacuating their children to Canada, that we wish to assist individually and collectively caring for these children. Those desiring to move children to Canada for duration of war, please contact us immediately. Will then arrange with Dominion Commission in placing children in suitable home environment."

After the Battle of Britain, the bombing of cities began. Both the

RCVS and the NVMA had moved precious records, portraits and the like from their London headquarters to less vulnerable places, so that the damage done to both premises was less traumatic than it might have been. The RCVS transferred its offices to Harrogate, and Council meetings were held in York.

*   *   *

John McFadyean died on the first day of February 1941, aged eighty-seven. A note at the end of a long obituary in *The Veterinary Record* said: "A full biography of Sir John McFadyean would entail the writing of the history of British veterinary science," a truth confirmed by repeated, but essential, reference to McFadyean in this short history of the profession. He was scientist, teacher, administrator, always a leader, incomparably the greatest veterinarian of his generation, whose pupils broadcast his professional wisdom and ideals. He was the last of the handful of great Victorian veterinary surgeons who fashioned the profession.

*   *   *

There have been few more desperate years in British history than 1941, yet those of privileged age recall the nation's determination to survive; not simply to continue to exist, but to create and enjoy a more generous world.

The Veterinary Record of 4th October 1941 looked to a future beyond war.

There would be great changes, it was said.

CHAPTER 20

Revolution in veterinary education — Veterinary Surgeons Act 1948

The changes forecast in 1941 were in veterinary education.

It will be recalled that veterinary research had been brought under the aegis of the Agricultural Research Council in the early 1930's, and that a State veterinary service, the Animal Health Division, had been established in 1938. Thus, only general practice and veterinary education remained outside the influence of Government. Practice being a private service between individuals was of no official concern, but the desirability of Government involvement in veterinary education was another matter.

In October 1936 the Minister of Agriculture and the Secretary of State for Scotland set up a committee: "To review the facilities available for veterinary education in Great Britain in relation to the probable future demand for qualified veterinary surgeons and to report thereon, and in particular to make recommendations as to the provisions which should be made from public funds in the five years 1937–42, in aid of the maintenance expenses of institutions providing veterinary education."

As originally constituted, only one of the five members of this committee was a veterinary surgeon (John Smith, recently elected to the Agricultural Research Council). *The Veterinary Record* of 31st October 1936 commented: "We cannot envisage any Government creating a similar committee of enquiry into medical education with but one medical representative out of five," and, under pressure from the NVMA, W.R. Wooldridge, Chairman of its Editorial Committee, was invited to serve. Thomas Loveday, Vice-Chancellor of Bristol University, was chairman. Presumably the reason for not including a representative of the RCVS, was that the committee was specifically charged with investigation of the finance of veterinary education, and it would have been inappropriate for the RCVS to be involved in voting public funds to support what had been its major preoccupation for ninety-four years.

The report of the Loveday Committee, summarised in *The Veterinary*

Record of 1st October 1938, said: "The whole lay-out of veterinary education is disjointed and unsystematic. A more organic connection is needed between the schools, the universities and the RCVS." There were numerous recommendations. Above all, and to the relief of those who had feared the worst, the single-portal of entry into the profession (corner-stone of RCVS policy since the 1844 Charter) was to be maintained. University involvement in veterinary education was strongly recommended. Students would acquire a degree, but there must in addition be acquisition of the RCVS diploma before they could practise as veterinary surgeons. The universities of Edinburgh, Glasgow, Liverpool, Cambridge, and London were recommended for location of veterinary schools, and "public funds should not be made available for veterinary teaching by any further universities." Emphasis was placed on the need for a field station, for practical instruction in animal husbandry, to be attached to each school. Salaries and status (including university professorships) of veterinary teachers should be improved. The capital investment would be £299,000, with recurring grants up to £61,000. There were numerous lesser recommendations, all favouring a more generous attitude towards the profession (with the possible exception of lady aspirants whose number "admitted by the schools should be small"). A new, but not unreasonable, concept was that: "The RCVS should be given power to include on its Council and Examination Committee representatives of the affiliated veterinary schools and of the five universities," a proposal nicely phrased to allow the RCVS to welcome, rather than unwillingly to accept, strangers at the Council table.

All in all, this Loveday report was a soothing document to a profession sensitive to outside pressure.

War intervened, however, and in September 1939 the report was shelved 'for the duration.'

There was surprise, therefore, when the Government recalled the Loveday Committee in February 1943, asking that the recommendations of 1938 be reviewed because of "great changes in the position and prospects of agriculture in this country." The reason for the resurrection of the Loveday Committee at this desperate time in a desperate war was that at high levels there had been a fundamental change in attitude to the veterinary profession. In 1938 veterinary surgeons were worthy fellows, to be encouraged as contributors to the Nation's wealth. In 1943 veterinary skill was vital if the people were to eat.

This change in image was born within the profession, through the NVMA Survey Scheme initiated in 1940, and the Veterinary Educational Trust set up in 1942 by NVMA President Wooldridge. Each of these enterprises was massively publicised, and each announced huge losses in milk and meat through animal disease.

Within a few months of the outbreak of war, an NVMA committee surveyed diseases of farm livestock, with a view to launching a co-ordinated attack by practising veterinary surgeons. Four diseases of cattle were specifically identified — mastitis, contagious abortion, Johne's disease, and infertility — and the operation to control them became known as the Survey Scheme. In an address to the 1940 NVMA Annual Meeting in Oxford, President Steele-Bodger said of the Survey Committee: "The fruits of its labours will, I believe, inaugurate a new charter for the Veterinary Profession . . . never was the time more propitious, never was it so necessary to avoid waste due to disease or indifferent animal husbandry."

The Scheme was developed with vigour by the NVMA, although some veterinary surgeons were embarrassed by the immense propaganda. The reason for their misgiving was that the diseases nominated for attack were poorly understood scientifically, and could *not* be eliminated, as might have been inferred from some of the more expansive statements. The most that could be achieved was a general improvement in husbandry through regular veterinary advice.

The publicity was a fact, however.

Describing foundation of the Veterinary Educational Trust, *The Daily Telegraph* of 30th September 1942 said: "Dr Wooldridge . . . estimated that 60 per cent of our dairy cattle were infected with one disease or another, and assessed at £50,000,000 annually the saving that would be achieved by what he called 'a bold co-ordinated animal health service.' "

Timing of the launch on 25th September 1942 of the Veterinary Educational Trust was psychologically perfect. War news was at its worst. The country ached for imaginative leadership in any field. The Trust was a new idea. An organisation to train the young, the deserving, the brilliant for research that would preserve Britain's livestock, second to none in the world. The Trust offered action *now*. As soon as money became available, scholarships and fellowships would be granted. The launching ceremony matched the magnitude of the task. A luncheon by courtesy of the Lord Mayor of the City of London at the Mansion House, was attended by some three hundred and fifty people, including Minister of Agriculture Hudson, each representing a well that could be tapped. The objective was £1,000,000 for the advancement of veterinary education. Success of the appeal was nationwide. The veterinary profession at once approved. The RCVS gave £1,000 and the NVMA £2,500. Within months the first Trust scholar had been selected.

The close relationship between the Loveday Committee and the Veterinary Educational Trust, was emphasised by the fact that of the six Committee members, five (Loveday, Barcroft, Burgess, Smith and Wooldridge) were on the Council of Management of the Trust.

The publicity thus created was not lost on a nation surrounded by submarines, but its consequence for the profession was unexpected. Having absorbed the fact of economic loss due to animal disease, the people asked: "How had this come about?" The answer was in the propaganda that created the question: "Because veterinary surgeons have not had the educational and research facilities required." Whose fault was this? Surely, said the people, the profession must be ineptly led?

In this manner a searchlight turned on the RCVS.

The Loveday Committee was recalled. Action was required. Legislation was expected.

The second Loveday report was published on 21st April 1944. It reinforced the first, but was more didactic towards the RCVS. Bristol University would be added to the five universities named in the first Report to provide veterinary education. The RCVS would remain the Governing Body of the profession, with power to inspect the university schools, but it must register university graduates as fit to practise, and must accept not only university but also Government representatives on its Council. There must be an immediate enquiry into unqualified practice, to precede any legislation that might arise from the report. Capital expenditure was estimated at £2,000,000, with £210,000 recurring annually.

Those who have followed this tale from its beginning, will realise the injustice of thus treating the RCVS as an erring infant. For precisely one hundred years it had struggled to create and to maintain a worthwhile profession. Time and time and time again it had sought, but had never found, support from Government. Now, when at last the profession's worth had by war been revealed, the indictment was that it had been inadequately led.

*   *   *

In the early 1940's there had been discussion among RCVS Councillors as to how the centenary of 1944 should be celebrated. The war had dampened enthusiasm, however, and no more ambitious suggestion had emerged than a commemorative booklet. Even this was set aside, however, when it was learned that *The Veterinary Record* would publish a comprehensive special number. The only RCVS centenary function in war-tormented 1944 was a luncheon at the Connaught Rooms, London, on 30th March, organised by the Central Veterinary Society.

To mark the occasion, President Hare of the Central Society presented to President Nairn of the RCVS an item of unusual interest. He said: "Like children all over the world, to find the wherewithal we ransacked the lumber room for bits and pieces long forgotten by our elders. We found, at least Jimmy found, a piece of the desk which belonged some 150 years ago to Principal Coleman. He also found the late Professor Penberthy's bloodstick, which is enclosed in a veterinary surgeon's instrument case. These relics have been fashioned by the craftsmanship of Hamilton Kirk into a President's gavel and stand."

In explanation: 'Jimmy' was Professor James McCunn of the London school. Hamilton Kirk was a practioner in London. A bloodstick was a short, thick-ended wooden stick, used in days gone by to tap a sharp triangular blade called a fleam into the jugular vein when a horse, or other large animal, was bled.

No record has been found of the menu for that luncheon. No doubt it included such war-time delicacies as dried-egg, spam, or snoek, but the dreariness of the food was forgotten in recalling great days, problems faced and battles won. There was another presentation — of the Central Society's cherished Victory Medal (commemorating the First World War) to RCVS Secretary Bullock. In his words of thanks, Fred Bullock matched the historic interest of the gavel and stand. He recalled that the Connaught Rooms, where he was speaking, occupied precisely the site of the Freemasons' Tavern where, on 12th April 1844, "the body politic and corporate of the Royal College of Veterinary Surgeons" met for the very first time.

An astonishing coincidence.

The centenary number of *The Veterinary Record* was dated 22nd December 1945, after the war had ended. The text had been ready for twelve months, but publication was delayed by printing difficulties and shortage of paper. The issue was edited by J.T. Edwards, whose interest in the history of the profession and whose close association with the *Record* from the time it was acquired by the NVMA, made this considerable undertaking a labour of love. It ran to some 100,000 words, spread over seventy-eight double-column pages of small print, and was crammed with information on all aspects of the profession. There were numerous contributors, covering the veterinary scene not only in Britain, but also in Eire, Canada, South Africa, India, New Zealand, Australia, and the non-self-governing dependencies.

*   *   *

The tribulations of life in war and the immediate post-war years are recalled by an advertisement in *The Veterinary Record* for 27th April 1946:-

> "Is there any member of the Association who has a Typewriter which he would be willing to sell to Headquarters? A 'Royal' would be preferable, but any make, however old, would be useful because it would be possible to exchange it. The staff is in urgent need of an extra machine and it is impossible to buy new or reconditioned models without waiting for many months."

It might have been supposed that such difficulties, multiplied a hundredfold in every aspect of living, would have delayed a Government response to the second Loveday Report. Not so. The recommendation that there be an enquiry into "the extent and effect of veterinary practice in Great Britain by persons who are not registered veterinary surgeons," was immediately implemented. A twelve-man committee under the chairmanship of Sir John Chancellor, and including Councillor P.J. Simpson representing the RCVS, and Sir Daniel Cabot, Chief Veterinary Officer of the Ministry of Agriculture and Fisheries, was set up within three months, and reported eight months later.

The veterinary profession was pleased with the recommendations of the Chancellor Committee. The two most important were that "practice of veterinary surgery by unregistered persons should be prohibited under penalty," and that persons "who for any seven of the preceding ten years have been engaged as their principal means of livelihood in diagnosing and giving medical or surgical treatment to animals," should be registered as "existing practitioners," and be subject to the disciplinary jurisdiction of the RCVS.

The road was now open for legislative implementation of the Loveday Report.

While the Chancellor Committee was deliberating (i.e. between July 1944 and March 1945), the RCVS Council discussed the Loveday recommendations. It would have been agreeable if their advice had been sought, and their experience tapped, but such courtesies were overlooked. The Councillors were under no illusion about being in the dock, and they acted with commendable pragmatism. They acted, too, with collective dignity inherited from their forefathers. Indeed, their position was remarkably similar to that of Thomas Turner and his Council in 1844, when Secretary Sir James Graham tried to steal back their Charter.

Dislike it more, or dislike it less, no one doubted that veterinary education was about to be changed, and that the major modification would be discontinuation of individual schools, in favour of integration within universities. No member of the RCVS Council objected to this principle. Indeed, they saw the advantages of better facilities and wider horizons as clearly as anyone. What they feared, however, was that the single portal of entry into the profession, that entailed passing a truly veterinary examination conducted by the RCVS, might be lost. If each university set its own standard and its own examination, uniformity in competence, especially in clinical subjects, would disappear. This point must be pressed hard with those on high.

In October 1944 the RCVS asked the Minister to convene a meeting of universities' representatives with the RCVS to discuss these points. Shortly afterwards, the RCVS received an unsolicited memorandum signed by some four hundred veterinary surgeons supporting the principle of veterinary education within universities, with safeguards to maintain the professional authority of the RCVS, and asking the RCVS to have discussions with "Responsible Authorities." The RCVS was reassured, therefore, that in already having opened negotiations, it was fulfilling the wishes of a significant proportion of the profession.

The unsatisfactory outcome of discussions between representatives of the Ministry of Agriculture, of the universities, and of the RCVS was reported to the RCVS Council late in April 1945. The universities had insisted that "if they were to interest themselves in veterinary education, they must be allowed to give a complete course with a degree which should be registrable as a qualification to practise."

This was the declaration that the RCVS had anticipated. In a letter of 1st May 1945 to the Minister, the position was made beyond peradventure clear. It was a splendid letter in the best RCVS tradition, signed by Secretary Bullock, the Minister's "obedient servant."

In measured paragraphs, it was emphasised that the RCVS Council was always anxious to improve veterinary education, and would be pleased to co-operate with universities to that end. It would be necessary, however, to have "power to send inspectors to report on the facilities at the Schools, the course of study and examinations, in the pre-clinical as well as the clinical years." Certain examination exemptions would be granted at certain schools in certain circumstances. There should be a trial period for this new system of veterinary education, and the RCVS "would endeavour to co-operate in as generous a spirit as possible." There was "no valid reason" why a university veterinary degree should be accepted by the RCVS "as a qualification to practise." Finally, the RCVS was "ready to co-operate to the fullest extent with the Universities short of giving up the right conferred on the College by its Charters and Statutes, namely, of deciding by its own Court of Examiners who are fit and proper persons to practise the Art and Science of Veterinary Medicine, Surgery and Obstetrics."

This letter contained the ingredients for any successful negotiation — a strong case presented with reason, firmness and courtesy. Minister Hudson did not reply in writing, but invited RCVS President Mitchell and "a few . . . friends" to an informal discussion on 7th June 1945. Notes were not taken of that meeting, but RCVS recollection was of reproving noises from the Minister in response to what was construed as intransigence.

There was then a pause in negotiations while Winston Churchill and Minister of Agriculture Hudson were replaced by Clement Attlee and Minister Williams.

A meeting between the RCVS and the new Minister was arranged for 28th November 1945. In preparation, the RCVS submitted a memorandum in which they asked: "In what respect is the Government dissatisfied with the professional ability of veterinary surgeons holding the Diploma of MRCVS?" Exception was taken, also, to Minister Hudson's statement that the Loveday Committee had been recalled "to prepare plans for effecting improvement in our National system of veterinary education, which is generally recognized to be necessary." The RCVS pointed out that as "the one body in the country which has made a special study of the subject" it had not been consulted.

At the meeting of 28th November, Minister Williams displayed political maturity by ignoring unanswerable criticism. Instead, with a welcoming smile, he said that "he had gone carefully over the field in consultation with the Secretary of State for Scotland and had reached the same conclusion as his predecessor, namely, that the proposals of the College did not provide for . . . essential needs . . . the recommendations of the Loveday Committee were strictly in line with modern educational opinion . . . he would be reluctant to do anything which would cause cleavage in the profession. He hoped, therefore, that the College would do their utmost to avoid such drastic action."

In transmitting a Draft Note of this meeting to Secretary Bullock of the RCVS, Secretary Hensley of the Ministry said that Minister Williams was anxious to announce to Parliament the intention of introducing legislation to (a) reconstitute the RCVS Council (b) give the RCVS powers to inspect veterinary teaching facilities and examinations in universities (c) after consultation with the Privy Council and the RCVS, authorize a university to grant a registrable veterinary degree (d) prevent veterinary practice by unqualified people.

These four points were debated by the RCVS Council on 10th January 1946. Councillors were agreed that they faced the inevitable, but if they co-operated with the Minister they would achieve, in essence, the standards they were seeking. Their greatest concession was reconstitution of the Council. Election to the RCVS Council was a coveted honour, an opportunity to contribute to the birth and growth of new ideas, to care for the profession. The prospect of having to discuss intimate veterinary matters with university and Government representatives who were not veterinary surgeons, however wise, raised no enthusiasm. Each point was discussed in turn and a vote taken, and in each case there was unanimous acceptance. In addition, it was agreed to implement immediately the Minister's suggestion to create an informal body of representatives of the RCVS, the existing schools, the universities to be involved, the Minister, and the Secretary of State for Scotland, to make plans for a future after legislation.

In a statement to Parliament on 1st April 1946, Minister Williams welcomed the recommendations of the Loveday and Chancellor Committees, and gave details of the four agreed principles on which it was "intended as soon as practicable to introduce legislation."

*   *   *

To the utmost regret of the veterinary world, RCVS Secretary Fred Bullock, LL.D, Barrister-at-Law, died on 14th February 1946, aged 67. In a memoir, RCVS President Mattinson wrote: "His relationship to us was unique; though not *de jure* one of the profession, he was *de facto* its very personification, and it is impossible to think of him as other than being 'one of us.' " Bullock's dedication to the profession was absolute. No task was too great, no day too long. He served the RCVS for thirty-nine years, that covered two great wars. His intense industry was matched by brilliant intellect. He was fluent in French, German, and Latin. His LL.D. thesis on "The Law Relating to Medical, Dental and Veterinary Practice" became a standard work. Every veterinary surgeon was grateful for his "Handbook" of 1927. His greatest love was the library that he cherished.

*   *   *

Strict confidentiality had to be maintained over negotiations towards legislation to cover the four proposals put to Parliament in April 1946 by Minister Williams. The veterinary profession knew nothing of continuous and complex discussions, until RCVS Secretary Oates, who had succeeded Bullock, was authorized to distribute copies of "Veterinary

Surgeons Bill 1948," together with explanatory notes. This document was undated, but was probably sent out about March 1948. It was followed by a memorandum, also undated, from RCVS President Dawes entitled: "Veterinary Surgeons Bill, 1948: Statement on the Progress of the Bill." This latter document referred to a meeting of the RCVS Council on 29th April 1948, and it was probably circulated to the profession shortly after that date.

It should have been clear to the profession that its interests had been well served. There should have been letters of congratulation on skilful compromise that had turned to the profession's advantage the enforced union with the universities. Instead, a critical storm was aimed at one item. The RCVS negotiators had had to agree that the unqualified people, whose livelihood during at least seven of the ten previous years had depended on treatment of sick animals, and who were to be taken on to a supplementary register and brought under RCVS discipline, should be designated "veterinary practitioners."

Typical letters to *The Veterinary Record* spoke of "great sadness and shame . . . because our leaders have apparently succumbed to intimidation," and of "the charlatan . . . at once given all the benefits enjoyed by us, after much toil and sweat." True, the Chancellor Committee had suggested the title "existing practitioner" for these unqualified people, as in the 1881 Act. However, in this case that title did not cover the clear precedent that a person who has earned his bread for a reasonable period in a specific and legal manner, must not be penalised when his occupation becomes the special privilege of a closed community and he himself becomes subject to the discipline of that community. He must be allowed a title that indicates his calling. Parliament was in no doubt about the justice of this decision, that so closely followed the Dentists Act of 1921 when qualified and unqualified men were, respectively, designated "dental surgeons" and "dentists." There would now be "veterinary surgeons" and "veterinary practitioners," otherwise there would be no Act. The matter was outside negotiation.

By contrast with the fuming over "veterinary practitioners," the concession of exemption of veterinary surgeons from jury service — a privilege repeatedly sought and refused for a hundred years — was barely noticed.

On 30th July the Act received the Royal Assent.

The Veterinary Surgeons Act of 1881 legalised the profession, and enabled the public to identify trained men. The Act of 1920 provided an income for the RCVS through an annual registration fee. The Act of

1948 brought education of the profession into the university system, and abolished unqualified practice.

Each was a bridge from an old world to a new, each a milestone on the veterinary journey.

Bibliography

From 1828 this history was based on page-by-page examination of veterinary journals, the first of which was published in that year. The high literary standard of the journals, and their comprehensive coverage of veterinary news, politics and science provided a detailed, and unbroken, account of development of the profession. The journals examined were:-

The Veterinarian (monthly) — 1828–1902

The Veterinary Journal (monthly) — 1875–1948 (still in publication as *The British Veterinary Journal*)

The Veterinary Record (weekly) — 1888–1948 (still in publication)

The Journal of Comparative Pathology & Therapeutics (quarterly) — 1888–1948 (still in publication as *The Journal of Comparative Pathology*)

Much information for the period 1791–1828 was obtained from:-

Pugh, L.P., 1962 *From Farriery To Veterinary Medicine: 1785–1795* Cambridge, W. Heffer & Sons.

Smith, F., 1976 *The Early History Of Veterinary Literature* London, J.A. Allen & Co. and Baillière, Tindall & Cox. Reprinted from various earlier sources.

Additional sources were:-

(A) *Archives* related to selected items generously made available by The Royal College of Veterinary Surgeons and the Royal Veterinary College, covering the whole period.

(B) *Documents* at the Public Record Office relating to cattle plague of 1865, kindly identified by the Librarian.

(C) *Publications*, as follows:-

Adami, Marie, 1930 *J. George Adami: A Memoir* London, Constable & Co.

Armatage, G., 1869 *The Thermometer As An Aid To Diagnosis In Veterinary Medicine* Leighton Buzzard, Muddiman.

Barlow, C. & P., 1971 *The Great Nobel Prizes: Robert Koch* London, Heron Books.

Blenkinsop, L.J. and Rainey, J.W., 1925 *History Of The Great War Based On Offical Documents: Veterinary Services* London, HMSO.

Bradley, O.C., 1923 *History Of The Edinburgh Veterinary College* Edinburgh & London, Oliver & Boyd.

Brock, T., 1961 *Milestones In Microbiology* Englewood Cliffs, N.J., U.S.A., Prentice-Hall, Inc..

Brooke, W.H., 1932 *Our Heraldry* Vet. Rec., *12*, 291.

Bulloch, W., 1938 *The History Of Bacteriology* Oxford, Oxford University Press.

Bullock, F., 1927 *Handbook For Veterinary Surgeons* London, Taylor & Francis.

Clabby, J., 1963 *The History Of The Royal Army Veterinary Corps* London, J.A. Allen & Co.

Clark, J., 1788 *A Treatise On The Prevention Of Diseases Incidental To Horses* Edinburgh, W. Smellie.

Coleman, E., 1796 *Instructions For The Use Of Farriers In Regiments Of Cavalry* London (No printer).

Cooper, B., 1843 *The Life Of Sir Astley Cooper, Bart.* London, John W. Parker.

D'Arcy Thompson, Ruth, 1974 *The Remarkable Gamgees* Edinburgh, The Ramsay Head Press.

Dick, W., 1869 *Occasional Papers On Veterinary Subjects* Edinburgh, William Blackwood & Sons.

Edinburgh Veterinary Review Edinburgh, Sutherland & Knox: London, Simpkin, Marshall & Co. Monthly: 1858–1864.

Farrier And Naturalist (later *Hippiatrist*) London. Published anonymously. Monthly: 1828–1830.

Gamgee, J., 1866 *The Cattle Plague* London, Robert Hardwicke.

Garnett, F.W., 1912 *Westmorland Agriculture 1800–1900* Kendal, Titus Wilson.

Great Britain, 1866 Commission on Cattle Plague. *First, Second And Third Reports Of The Commissioners Appointed To Inquire Into The Origin And Nature Of Cattle Plague, 1865–1866* London, HMSO.

Great Britain, 1868 Veterinary Department. *Report On The Cattle Plague In Great Britain During The Years 1865, 1866 And 1867. Appendix II Medical Report By Professors Simonds And Brown* London, HMSO.

Great Britain, 1922 Development Commission. Advisory Committee on Research into Diseases of Animals. *Report Of The Advisory*

Committee On Research Into Diseases Of Animals London, HMSO. (The Prain Report).

Great Britain, 1929 Committee on the Colonial Veterinary Service. *Report On Veterinary Research And Administration In The Colonies* London, HMSO. (The Lovat Report).

Great Britain, 1929 Committee on the Reconstruction of the Royal Veterinary College. *Report Of The Departmental Committee On The Reconstruction Of The Royal Veterinary College* London, HMSO. (The Martin Report).

Great Britain, 1938 Ministry of Agriculture and Fisheries & Department of Agriculture for Scotland. *Report Of The Committee On Veterinary Education In Great Britain* London, HMSO. (The Loveday Report).

Great Britain, 1944 Ministry of Agriculture and Fisheries & Department of Agriculture for Scotland. *Second Report Of The Committee On Veterinary Education In Great Britain* London, HMSO. (The Second Loveday Report).

Great Britain, 1965 Ministry of Agriculture, Fisheries and Food. *Animal Health A Centenary: 1865-1965* London, HMSO.

Hall, S.A., 1962 *The Cattle Plague Of 1865 Med. Hist.*, 6, 45.

Hall, S.A., 1965 *John Gamgee And The Edinburgh New Veterinary College Vet. Rec.*, 77, 1237.

Jones, A., 1933 *Memoirs Of A Soldier Artist* London, Stanley Paul & Co.

Journal Of The Royal Agricultural Society Of England London. Published by the Society. 1840-still in publication.

Keynes, G., 1966 *The Life Of William Harvey* Oxford, Clarendon Press.

Noble, W.C., 1974 *Leonard Colebrook* London, W. Heinemann.

Pattison, I., 1980 *William Hunting's Birthday Vet. Rec.*, 107, 578.

Pattison, I., 1981 *The Veterinary Surgeons Act, 1881 Vet. Rec.*, 108, 157.

Pattison, I., 1981 *John McFadyean: A Great British Veterinarian* London & New York, J.A. Allen & Co.

Simonds, J.B., 1894 *Autobiography* Reprinted from *The Veterinarian* London, Adlard & Son.

Simonds, J.B., 1896 *Biographical Sketch Of Delabere P. Blaine And William Youatt* London, Adlard & Son.

Simonds, J.B., 1897 *The Foundation Of The Royal Veterinary College With Biographical Sketches Of St Bel, Edward Coleman, William Sewell And Charles Spooner* London, Adlard & Son.

Simonds, J.B., 1898 *A Biographical Sketch Of William John Thomas Morton* London, Adlard & Son.

Smith, F., 1927 *A History Of The Royal Army Veterinary Corps:*

1796–1919 London, Baillière, Tindall & Cox.

Walley, T., 1890 *A Practical Guide To Meat Inspection* Edinburgh & London, Young J. Pentland.

Wilson, G.S., 1979 *The Brown Animal Sanatory Institution J. Hyg. Camb.*, *82*, 155, 337, 501: *83*, 171.

Index